AF885140

Olanzapine Psychopathological and Psychopharmacological Indications and Possibilities

by Hajime Jozuka, M. D.
Department of Psychiatry & Psychosomatic Medicine
Jozuka Mental Clinic & JMC Stress Medical Institute

Copyright © 2011 by Hajime Jozuka, M.D.

All rights reserved, including the right to reproduce this book or portions thereof in any form whatsoever, without the express written consent of the author.

ISBN 978-0-9833352-2-1

Biblio Books

Dedicated to
all patients
everywhere

Abstract

Olanzapine has been considered a drug for the treatment of schizophrenic disorders and bipolar disorders, but only this drug among the antipsychotics operates selectively on A10 nerves. As a result, it is legal to prescribe this drug for only a narrow range of symptoms and for very few diseases.

The retrospective research described in this book was performed on 453 patients who improved remarkably from Olanzapine. The 453 patients are classified as follows: 54 Olanzapine patients at the last prescription, 50 patients on Olanzapine and other major antipsychotics, 90 patients on selective serotonin reuptake inhibitors (SSRIs), 42 on SSRIs and 42 on Olanzapine from the first to last prescription, and 42 on Olanzapine and Ariprazol. The results showed that 286 patients improved with only Olanzapine. Furthermore, it was suspected that Olanzapine contributed to the elevation of both the T-cell system and natural-killer cell activity. The conclusions suggested that Olanzapine can contribute to the amelioration and/or cure of many other diseases.

Table of Contents

Preface

Since the beginning of the 21st century, new antipsychotic drugs, called atypical antipsychotics, have become available, one after another. Furthermore, as each medicine has appeared on the market, it has been considered sufficient. In other words, it is generally held that one specific antipsychotic drug is sufficient and is effective to treat psychoses, especially schizophrenia. On the one hand, this mono-medication approach would be easy to effect because not only experienced psychiatrists, but any beginner psychiatrist, even a psychiatric resident, would be qualified to prescribe long-term use of the drug. In addition, if schizophrenia were improved by only one medicine, the quality of life (QOL) of schizophrenic patients would rapidly improve. However, such a simple solution has never enjoyed enduring success throughout the history of psychiatry. Unfortunately, hope is not the same as fact.

Nevertheless, as psychopharmacology has developed over the years, the hope has gradually grown closer to the facts and actions in medical history. Furthermore, as brain science has grown and developed, the function of the A10 nerves—and the relationship between A10 nerves and the peripheral areas—have been clarified.

After the demise of psychiatry in some developed countries, psychopathological considerations began to resurface in core psychiatry. Along with this development, medical anthropological studies—not cognitive scientific research—gradually gained favor in the discipline of psychiatry, and revolutionary phenomena have increased, especially in psychopharmacology. In this atmosphere, there has been a rediscovery of the effects of Olanzapine.

The medicine had been prescribed only as a schizophrenia-indicative medicine, but it was discovered that the medicine has a selective impact on the A10 nerve function. This fact indicates that the medicine has an effect on the human personality.

As a result of these discoveries, there has been a flurry of research about Olanzapine.

In this book, I describe many other indications and possibilities for Olanzapine by virture of clinical experiments.

Olanzapine is not indicative for schizophrenia alone, but for many other situations, as well.

Chapter I: Introduction

Early on, I noticed that a prescription of Olanzapine is not officially permitted only for schizophrenia and bipolar disorders in Japan, although Olanzapine is legally prescribed for other diseases in many countries.

In fact, Olanzapine is often prescribed for assorted diseases, although such prescriptions are officially prohibited, for reasons of effectiveness and safety. And this could well be the case in other countries. Some drugs that are actually dangerous are liberally prescribed in some countries, including Japan, to avoid lawsuits or to stay within the law.

When the psychopathological and psychopharmacological studies on schizophrenia and its associated disorders—and also on chronic mental disorders—were investigated, some interesting results came to light. The stories of some of these studies will be described in this book.

Although the existence of schizophrenia has been well known, and psychopathological studies have been conducted for many years, the true character of schizophrenia has never been defined or agreed upon in the collective view, even until today.(4)(12)-(20)

Martin Heidegger defined a human being philosophically and psychopathologically as a "spatiotemporal life order," and he defined disease as a "crisis of the life order." His definition succeeded the works of Binswanger, von Weiztsaecker, Boss, and Kimura, but it seems curious that there is no collective view on schizophrenia. Although a substantive definition of schizophrenia has never been clarified, it seems very strange that many drugs, which are shown to have an effect on schizophrenia, have been made and prescribed for many years, up through the present.(4)(12)-(24) As a result, I have arrived to the conclusion that the object of the drugs known as antipsychotics might actually be atypical psychosis or schizoaffective disorder instead of schizophrenia.

In fact, although innumerable psychopathological and psychobiological studies on atypical psychosis or schizoaffective disorder have been developed, no drug to treat these illnesses has been available and approved in the history of psychiatry. I find it profoundly strange that this is the case, and that the situation will probably continue into the future.

Considering these phenomena, I cannot help nourishing a suspicion that nearly all psychiatrists who diagnose schizophrenia by using a symtomatic manual made in the United States, have actually treated only atypical psychosis or schizoaffective disorder because it is not possible to diagnose schizophrenia by symptoms or symptomatology. And, since it is virtually impossible to diagnose schizophrenia by use of symptomatic manual books, these doctors might be treating only atypical psychosis or schizoaffective psychosis, including schizophrenia.

In this connection, no diagnostic manual has been written about non-symptomatic schizophrenia (or kernel schizophrenia) (Die Kern-schizophrenia)(12)-(24). It is well known that schizoaffective disorder, which has been symptomatically defined in the Diagnostic and Statistical Manual of Mental Disorders, 3rd. Edition (DSM-III), has never been treated with any drug in psychopharmacological history until recently. In fact, this disorder has been treated by officially illegal drugs.

Schizoaffective disorder, as a symptomatic diagnosis, has been called and treated psychopathologically as an atypical psychosis ever since this disorder was defined as a schizoaffective disorder by DSM-III(1) over 20 years ago. At first, this disorder was called—and treated as—Zykloide Psychose, Episodische Catatonia, or acute schizoaffective psychosis. As a result, two opinions emerged: 1. the disorder was treated as an independent condition, and 2. it was treated as a special kind of schizophrenia.

From then on, the disorder has been treated on an individual basis, but Pauleikhoff, B., Hatotani, T. and others clarified and defined the atypical psychosis or schizoaffective psychosis as a biological psychosis.(2)(3) The common characteristics of the diseases that they defined are:

1. Onset is acute; the prognosis is good at each occurrence, but the disease has a tendency to recur.
2. Dominated by emotion, consciousness and psychomotoric disorders.
3. Over time, bipolarity in symptoms like manic-depressive, anxiety-trance and excitement-confusion are observed.
4. When an attempt was made to find conclusions based on these phenomena (although a biological basis has never been established for the psychosis called schizophrenia), some biologists defined schizophrenia as a biological disorder and condition.(4)

As a result, a number of psychiatrists began to consider treating it with pharmacotherapy. This is the case even until now, and it is astonishing how many antipsychotics have been developed and produced for the psychosis. It would seem that all this ushered in an era defined by "keeping up with the times."

Although clinicians have been eagerly awaiting new effective drugs to treat patients on an ongoing basis, unfortunately these antipsychotics (called atypical antipsychotics, whose common names are Quetiepine, Risperidon, Perospirone, Olanzapine, Aripirazol, Pronanceline, Bespirone, etc.) have not provided remarkable effects for patients, except for slightly reduced side effects and slightly increased safety factors, compared with the former traditional antipsychotics.

Chapter II: The New Atypical Antipsychotics

Conventional thinking has held that there *is* no special atypical antipsychotic that is effective. Fortunately, it was finally recognized that there is one effective atypical antipsychotic agent—Olanzapine. The special feature of Olanzapine is that it operates selectively on A10 nerves, which have been thought to preside over the integration of the human brain. Some drugs that operate on A9 nerves have been available, but until recently, there has been no drug that operates exclusively on the A10 nerves, which is a nonaggressive area because A10 nerves have to do with human character and personality. At last, recent studies and reports(5)-(8) show that Olanzapine operates selectively. It would not be overstating the case to say that there has never been a drug that is more effective than Olanzapine because no other drug has been shown to have an exact selective operation on the A10 nerves.

The A10 nerves in the tegmentum of the midbrain are connected with the midbrain amygdaloidal nucleus (related to emotion, fear, adaptability), hippocampus and basal ganglia (related to somatic motor), nucleus accumbens (related to the limbic system, known as the emotional and visceral brain) and the frontal association area (related to personality, movement motivation and planning). And it secrets Dopamine, which promotes awareness of pleasure.

The amygdaloidal nucleus assesses an individual's likes and dislikes, and the basal ganglia express the result of these assessments through the face muscles. The nucleus accumbens promotes volition, and the fovea cortex promotes feelings of well being and intellectual good feeling in the frontal association area, which secrets twice the usual Dopamine during periods of well being.

Recently, there is speculation that the A10 nerves actually work as the conductor in the overall brain.

Figure 1, below, shows the anatomy of the A10 nerves and the Neurotransmission Systems.(29)-(32)

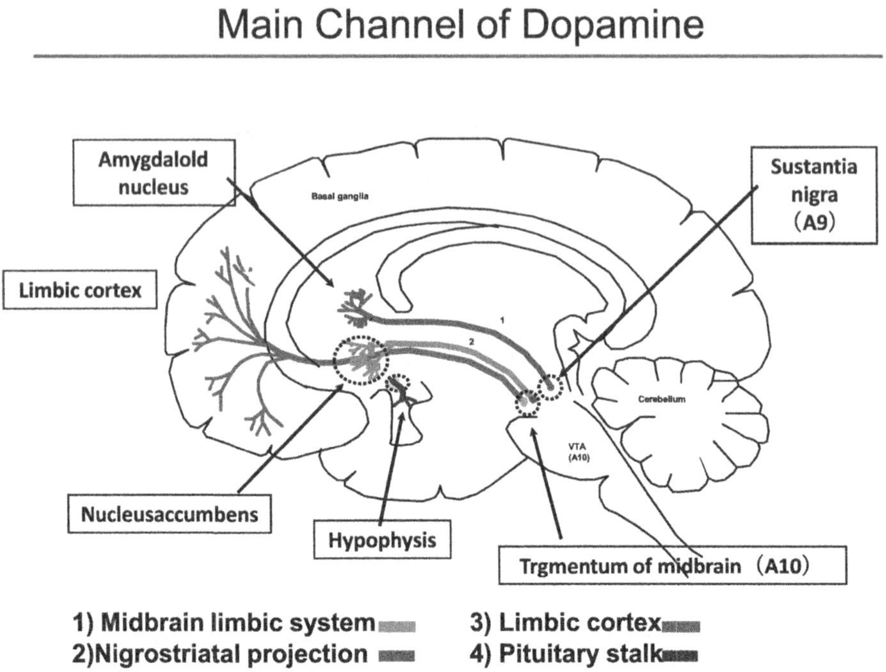

Figure 1: Anatomy of A10 Nerve and Neurotransmission Systems

It is commonly known that there are conditions too numerous to mention called and diagnosed as schizoaffective disorder or atypical psychoses. Mecical history is full of these phenomena.

Fortunately, as I have mentioned, schizoaffective disorder has been studied under several names and conditions before the name was defined by DSM-III. For example: Zykloide Psychose, Episodische Catatonia and acute schizoaffective psychosis.(3)

With the appearance of Olanzapine, certain conditions and situations of diseases are thought to be Olanzapine effective. These are described in Figure 2., below.(9)

[Sensory deprivation phenomena: acute traumatic psychosis, prison psychosis, cerebrovascular disorders, dementia]
[Drug dependence and alcoholism including withdrawal symptoms]
[Symptomatic psychoses: diabetic psychotics, hyperthyroidism, brain tumor]
[Symptomatic psychoses: viral or bacterial encephalitis]
[Latrogenic psychoses: post-operative psychosis, ICU psychoses, hemodialysis psychosis]
[SLE psychosis] etc.
⇓ ⇓
[Schizoaffective disorder or atypical psychoses]

Figure 2: Diseases and symptom groups showing schizoaffective disorder or atypical psychoses.

It might be thought that these disease groups (either suddenly or gradually) extend to inclusion in matters of missing brain integration, and express as psychoses due to similar somatic or biological problems, although the original diseases differ from each other. For example, it is thought that diabetes psychotics involves symptoms such as falling in confusion and disability of brain integration, due to the predictable incorrect glucose thickness in the brain because of the instability of serum glucose thickness in diabetes mellitus. In such a situation, Olanzapine could have a precise effect, since the drug takes part in glucose metabolism.(9) And I believe that any effect thought to be a side effect would have to be reevaluated as a desired effect. However, the prescription of Olanzapine for diabetes mellitus is officially prohibited in Japan.

It is well known that any human being will fall into sensory deprivation in a situation such as the following: A person, who has been rushing from place to place suddenly meets with a traffic accident and suffers a fracture of the cervical vertebra. He will, unfortunately, be forced into complete bed rest; he will have to be still and look at a white ceiling all day long, although—prior to the accident—he lived a very stimulating life, involved with his friends, listening to interesting music, reading books, and enjoying nature. Then, suddenly, he has to live in bed without stimulation and without permission to move, except only to look at the white ceiling. If such a situation continues for several hours to several days, the patient will begin to feel as if the white ceiling is moving on both sides; he may perceive that the ceiling is crawling with many small worms. He will be terrified, or suddenly get angry and excitable. Sometimes he may start to behave violently.

In a situation like this, nearly all brain function becomes disconnected and loses its so-called integration.

Such acute derangement has been treated by major tranquilizers like Haloperidol, but this drug is more dangerous for patients. Since safety is an issue, a drug like Olanzapine, which is immediately effective and which is safe, should be prescribed; it should be the drug of first choice in such cases. And since sensory-deprivation phenomena are common, not only in acute traumatic psychosis, but also in prison psychosis, cerebra-vascular disorders, and night delirium of dementia, their situations, including withdrawal symptoms because of drug dependence and alcoholism, raise the same or similar pathological mechanisms.

Olanzapine is the only reasonable choice for effectiveness because only Olanzapine operates on the A10 nerves, while other drugs operate only on the nerve groups through A9.(5)-(8)

Additional symptomatic psychoses are shown in Figure 3 below.

[Depressions]→[Deterioration of Typus Melencholicus Depression, Exhausted Type Depression & Anxiety Disorder]
[Sichizoaffectic Disorder (schizophrenic disorder-like situations)] → [PTSD]
[Exhaustic Psychoses] →[CFS]
[Borderline Personality Disorders] →[Re-integration of Personality by A10 operation]

CF: PTSD: Psychotraumatic stress disorder, CFS: Chronic fatigue syndrome

Figure 3: Olanzapine Effective Diseases—invited after symptomatic diseases as selective operative A10-nerves drug

These psychoses are described as exhausted psychosomatics, mental integration disorder, and lack of personality integration.

Depression of Typus Melancholicus, which has been psychopathologically emphasized, should be enumerated in these situations since the first victims of Typus Melancholicus are thought to be so seriously attached to a sense of order that they will go to the length of self-sacrifice to protect that order.(11) Tellenbach, H. has argued that this Typus Melancholicus is a psychopathological feature peculiar to the Japanese, but he has overlooked a psychopathologically more fundamental feature: if Typus Melancholicus is based on an attachment to order, and if it has existed until today, there should be some inherent basis for this in the Japanese people. One could make a case that the origin is in the spirit of Confucianism, which has not been mentioned since the end of World War II. Instead, as the current thinking goes, the simple existence of the Japanese people has succeeded Confucianism.

Although Confucianism harkens to the Fifth Century, it was completely generalized after the end of the Nineteenth Century (known as Meiji-time). Confucianism had sustained the fundamental spirituality of the Japanese people until the end of World War II, when prohibition of traditional ideas was imposed. But this spirit has continued to exist in the psychological depths of the people, though it has gradually changed into a contemporary attachment to order because of the denial of the ideas of Confucianism.

On the other hand, since the Japanese government began to suppress traditional ideas as the national administrative policy from the 1970s, Typus Melancholicus-type depression has gradually decreased in the population. Afterwards, the Japanese people (those who were educated about the denial of traditional ideas in their adolescence in the 1970s), grew up and produced a generation of children whose ideas are confused. As a result, chronic fatigue syndrome and borderline personality disorders have increased, along with a decrease in Typus Melancholicus-type depression.

Since exhausted depressions were readily found among sufferers of psychopathological problems, such patients were treated with selective serotonin re-uptake inhibitors (SSRIs), along with supportive psychotherapy. In fact, these patients were able to return to their normal lives in as little as six months. Unfortunately, it has never been recognized that the diseases mentioned above are deep pathologically exhaustive diseases. As a result, treatments are tried and continued for long periods of time while doctors wait to discover if there has been improvement, so recovery can take a very long time.

These kinds of situations are specific to the Japanese people. As a result, it could be assumed that Japanese depression and other disorders would not be treatable using symptomatic diagnostic definitions formulated in the United States. In other words, major depression in the Fourth Edition of the Diagnostic and Statistical Manual of Mental Disorders, 4th. Ed. (DSM-IV-TR) fundamentally differ from Japanese depression, which is often based on the attachment of the Japanese to order. Japanese depression would not be treatable with SSRIs. Instead, Japanese depression would have to be treated with A10 nerve operative agents. SSRIs, as well as serotonin and epinephrine reuptake inhibitors (SNRIs) might be effective for major depression diagnosed by symptomatically diagnostic manuals, but might not be effective for depression based on deep psychopathological problems.

The recent generation of psychiatrists tends to diagnose and treat not only depression but also other psychotic diseases by using symptomatic diagnostic manuals without taking into account the individual psychopathology of each client. What's more, many of these practitioners do not understand the syndrome that I call "attachment to order" that is prevalent in the Japanese population. It is unfortunate that many psychiatrists today do not recognize the deep psychopathological problems underlying mental disorders, including depression. Even though more and more effective antidepressant agents have been developed, suicide rates have seriously increased.

It is thought that exhaustive depressions should be treated first by improving the exhaustion of the patient, and then the corresponding socially depressive mood. From this point of view, I suspect that the suitability of Olanzapine will spread and will result in a formula such as the following: Rest→Recovery of Integration→Improvement of Depression.

There is speculation that the behavior of Dopamine and Serotonin, as well as selective operations of the A10 nerves will respond to this medication in a way that the effectiveness of the medication is elevated.

When psychopathology is considered, depressions of typus melancholicus are never confused with contemporary depression known as major depression. Thus, I ventured to describe these depressions as depression of typus melancholicus, in spite of major depression.

When depression is diagnosed in transcultural psychiatry, depression of typus melancholicus fundamentally differs from major depression in DSM-IV-TR.

Psycho-Traumatic Stress Disorder

It might naturally occur that both the exhausted depressions and the worse anxiety disorders arise from the same pathological situations. In this connection, psycho-traumatic stress disorder (PTSD) and the Japanese "attachment to order" syndrome could evolve from a common fundamental psychopathogenesis. As a result, Japanese PTSD extends over a long period of time because the current ongoing political and social climate in Japan encourages destruction of (not attachment to) order. Consequently, it is possible that even a symptomatically defined diagnosis of psycho-traumatic stress disorder may not be acclimatized to Japanese people.

An individual Japanese patient of PTSD might suffer not only as the victim of the destruction of order, but also as the destroyer himself—not only of his personal order, but also the order of his peripheral society. This patient may not recognize himself as a victim or as an assailant; or even that he is involved in this phenomenon. His ideation might be the same as the ideation of typus melancholicus depression, and his condition might be "post festum" (after the festival). Since he will have to live in a retrieval situation and situations and society, it will be natural that his pathological condition extends over a long period of time. Although he will live by a survival instinct, sometime his lifestyle will be similar to schizophrenia due to disturbed brain integration. It is quite possibly a common phenomenon, if we were to re-read the history sheet, that although a person was treated as a PTSD patient at the first visit, he will be treated as a schizophrenic afterwards.

To my surprise, PTSD victims, in most cases, do not respond to antidepressants, despite symptoms of depression and anxiety. For such cases, however, Olanzapine offers some important possibilities, since—in such situations—it relieves pain and integrates spirit.

Chronic Fatigue Syndrome

In cases of chronic fatigue syndrome (CFS), it is well known that ordinary clinics often misdiagnose the disorder as intractable depression. As a result, such patients are treated with a variety of antidepressants and supportive psychotherapy over long periods of time. Of course, they do not improve and sometimes, they end up being hospitalized. When exhaustion is discovered in such patients, strict rest is prescribed. But, it is commonly known that patients suffering from CFS complain that they are usually unaware of or don't experience feelings of exhaustion, which indicates a disturbance of the A10 nerves. Furthermore, these patients usually try to continue their routines, including jogging and other strenuous activity, despite of serious muscle pain.

The underlying issues in CFS are the precise opposite of those in typus melancholicus. The fact is that psychotherapies are never effective for CFS sufferers. Since they are generally and completely exhausted (even though they often feel no exhaustion), it is suspected that their brains may lack integration. When they are treated with psychotherapy, they sometimes are forced to feel something that they are actually not experiencing. CFS patients should be treated with medication that will allow them to rest. And Olanzapine could be the most effective agent against CSF. It is likely to allow patients to experience their exhaustion and to give them rest from it by the effect of brain integration.

CFS patients often conform to a type-A behavior pattern, which is defined as a mental and external personality that is impetuous, workaholic, and persistent. Such personalities are often unmanageable and often feel hatred toward others. The distinctive CFS personality could be thought of in terms of the "crisis of life order" personality in Heidegger's Theory.(46)

There is speculation that CFS results from the raising (by the patient) of self-integrative incontinentia, because the prognostic situation is similar to schizophrenia. At first, patients suffering from CFS with serious exhaustion—like patients suffering serious depression—are treated with the usual methods, but they do not show positive response to the treatments and, over time, they fall into a desolation of spirit and a personality. Although at first, the CFS sufferer seems to be an able person, at the last analysis, CFS is similar to schizophrenia in the desolation of spirit and social experiences.

If this speculation were commonly recognized, it might not seem strange for Olanzapine to be the medication of choice in treating CFS. Because CFS would come to be regarded as similar to schizophrenia, it would be commonly treated in a similar way.

Olanzapine could well have astonishing effects for these patients. It could improve the condition and shorten the time until remission. In other words, the fovea cortex in the A10 nerves can be confused in CFS patients, which renders them unable to feel a common sense of well being. It is possible that the re-integration of the operation of the A10 nerves is effected by Olanzapine, not Dopamine and Serotonin. Olanzapine should be selected as the drug of choice for CFS.

Borderline Personality Disorders

Borderline personality disorders (BPD) are characterized by antisocialism, selfishness, emotional instability and the coexistence of the so-called angelic personality and devilish personality. Much has been written about sufferers of this disorder. They can appear to be very socially skilled, then suddenly the antisocial side takes over. They can become violent and even commit murder for no apparent reason. Olanzapine should be prescribed for borderline personality disorder.(58)-(67)

When Olanzapine—along with psychotherapy—is prescribed immediately after diagnosis of borderline personality disorders, within a short time, socialization is possible, with long-term success rates. This phenomenon has been observed in many countries, not only in Japan.

Psychopharmacologically, this phenomenon can be explained in terms of the effect that Olanzapine has on Dopamine operation. Olanzapine promotes the predominant assertion of Dopamine, which then operates selectively on the A10 nerves, enabling a borderline personality to re-integrated into a normal situation.

Olanzapine—accompanied by a special psychotherapy and some behavioral therapies—is commonly prescribed as the drug of choice. In cases where Olanzapine alone was not effective, Olanzapine(5mg/day) plus Aripirazol (3mg/day) can elevate the effect, or Aripirazol (6mg/day) alone. Schizophrenic disorders are officially treated with Olanzapine as the last. These ideas may not be officially recognized, and they may not to be in proper historical order, but the biological details of schizophrenia have never been decisively clarified.

Furthermore, when I consider the psychopathological studies that have been done on schizophrenia, I see that nearly all opinions resulting from these studies remain in the context of "stress functional disorder in life history" and "biopathological change" theories.(4)(10)

I recognize that the actual problem that "positive symptoms," which were commonly regarded as mark symptoms in the early studies, differ from schizoaffective disorders, and so are gradually developing delusional-hallucinogenic situations. It is thought that when these situations are left untreated for long periods of time, then delusional-hallucinogenic situations would become a permanent and irreversible biological change.(4) (12)-(24)

But, so called "negative symptoms" are psychopathologically considered and defined as "the core of schizophrenia itself," although it has never been clarified what kind of situation this is by any developer of Olanzapine.

I cannot be other than skeptical about a situation that is called a "schizophrenic disorder," but whose symptoms are not uniformly recognized in the field and it is an obscure syndrome, and has been misunderstood in the treatment history of psychiatry.

The schizophrenic disorder, as defined in DSM-III, was thought not to be an individual disease. The schizophrenic disorder was defined as the syndrome, about which Dr. Robert L. Spitzer, one of editors of DSM-III, had emphasized, saying that these disorders (found in DSM-III) are persistently the maximum common divisors to be recognized by all specialists. Of course, however, these syndromes have never been conclusively defined as a single disease.(1)

Unfortunately, there exist some strange phenomena in the field of psychiatry. For instance, many specialists are diagnosing and treating patients based on only DSM-IV-TR. In other words, I recognize that misunderstandings, and resulting misdiagnoses and treatments, could be due to the common opinion that non-specific schizophrenia exists, in spite of the existence of a precise diagnosis for schizophrenia by DSM-IV-TR. However, DSM-IV-TR is not universally recognized. It has been said that this symptomatic and statistical manual was made for the purpose of discussing all psychotic disorders at the same table. But its contents are still fluid.

It should be recognized that schizophrenia based on DSM-IV-TR might not exist, and that schizophrenia based on the diagnoses of a particular specialist might indeed exist. We must conclude that many specialists diagnose and treat patients suffering from schizophrenia based on psychopathology, and that this is fundamentally different from schizophrenia based on DSM-IV-TR.

It is easy to perform statistical research on schizophrenia as defined by the DSM-IV-TR. Unfortunately, such a manual is not always useful for clinical specialists, who are working with actual human beings with all their complexities and using practical treatments.

This kind of situation could invite the collapse of psychiatry in the United States. Avoidance and denial of psychotherapy as a valid approach has already become common among specialists. It is possible that cognitive-behavioral scientific orientations are taking the place of traditional psychiatry and psychology, according to *Nature*, an American publication.

The most important and significant process in psychoanalytic therapies was traditionally to listen quietly to clients' descriptions of their situations and complaints over a long period, and to accept their psychopathological and psycho-physiological situations. Through these therapies, clients will unconsciously elevate their psycho-physiology and acceptably integrate their psychopathological problems.

In the history of psychotherapy, therapists in the United States have gradually changed approach to what I consider wrong therapeutic methods: the therapist directly informs the client of the relationship between the symptoms the client is feeling now (usually pain) and a psychopathological problem, which the patient had experienced a long time ago. For example, a therapist might tell a patient that the symptom he or she is experiencing has to do with an experience of sexual cruelty in adolescence—and that he cannot change this fact, but must learn to accept it. When the patient is abruptly made aware of this kind of unfortunate fact, which he had already forgotten, he can easily fall into a depressive state and can even (as commonly occurs) become suicidal.

As a result, clients who are weak and vulnerable come to curse their past experiences and fall into a state of denial of themselves in the present and future. In such situations, clients often come to accuse their psychoanalysts, due to a perception of having lost their future. Needless to say, one peripheral result is an increase in lawsuits, since clients pay a lot of money to therapists in United States.

It might not be too much of a stretch to say that Japanese psychiatry, which has (superficially, at least) copied trends from the U.S., would also collapse in such a manner. Already, many Japanese psychiatric specialists have relegated psychotherapies, including psychoanalysis, to the dustbin of the past. In my judgment, they are avoiding their responsibility in the clinical setting by inviting the cognitive/behavioral science as a replacement.

Psychoanalytic methods and other psychotherapies have already moved away from the original models, for example, Freud, S. and Jung. C.G. in the U.S. and Japan. Nearly all psychiatrists and psychologists have selected new methods based on cognitive behavioral sciences. And spiritual science has begun to collapse in the United States, as well. With the establishment of the cognitive/behavioral science, therapists have forgotten the relationship between spirit and mind. The idea that mind is separate from heart and spirit has already become entrenched in scientific thinking.

Therapists who try to use psychoanalytic and psycho-spiritual therapies, are an endangered species in the U.S., so a natural spiritual as well as mental relationship between client and therapist is disappearing in psychiatric treatments in the U.S.—and in Japan, too, where the landscape is looking much like American escape theory. It should hardly be worthwhile to learn from psychiatrists in the U.S., but it appears that many Japanese psychiatrists wish to fall into step with the U.S.

They have forgotten the Japanese psychiatrist, Morita, M., who already established the cognitive behavioral science, called "Morita Therapy," in the history of Japanese psychiatry. Morita Therapy was based on cognitive behavioral science. Contemporary Japanese psychiatrists have imported Americanized Japanese cognitive behavioral science without awareness of the re-import.

In the next chapters, I will put forward studies based on the precise psychopathological studies and results and not be limited by these practices.

Chapter III: Clinical Studies on Olanzapine

Background

In situations such as those described in the previous chapters, I have experience with, and have treated, many psychotic clients who have never been clearly diagnosed with schizophrenia or bipolar disorder. In other words, I have seen many patients who were given such psychopathological diagnoses as schizophrenia; but who were not diagnosed as schizophrenia according to the DSM-IV-TR. These patients never showed any improvement from officially permitted medications. Olanzapine is the only medication, in my experience, that has afforded improvement to schizophrenic patients with psychopathological diagnoses.

Of course, I have consistently recognized that DSM-IV-TR has been the foundation of clinical diagnoses in nearly all countries. Nevertheless, Olanzapine is the medication that has provided significant and consistent improvement for clients who were not diagnosed as schizophrenic in DSM-IV-TR.

In the following pages, I will introduce descriptions and discussion of some of these cases.

The research in these studies was performed retrospectively and conducted in strict accordance with the Ethical Code. The studies were "client centered" and the interviews and analyses took place in my clinic.

Subjects & Methods

Subjects

The subjects were 453 cases who were treated at the Department of Psychiatry in the Jozuka Mental Clinic in Nishio, Aichi Japan for three consecutive years. All of 453 cases were prescribed Olanzapine.

Methods

The investigations on the effects and transitions of the prescription were performed retrospectively in order to exclude any intention from the therapist.

These investigations were performed on the relationships between and among SSRIs, Aripirazol (switching from Olanzapine) and Olanzapine.

Although these subjects were treated as though they had been diagnosed by use of DSM-IV-TR—using officially permitted medications at the beginning of the treatment—they never showed improvement. Some did show changes for the worse, however. All subjects improved dramatically with Olanzapine under the psychopathological diagnosis "schizophrenia," after going through changes of medication over time.

In this connection, the Association of Ethics holds that only the last diagnoses should be expressed; other detail drugs should not be described because individual privacy might be specified.

Therefore, only main drugs are shown in Figure 4, below.

The research was undertaken to investigate histories of prescription from the first medication to the last medication, retrospectively, in three groups as follows: (1) groups of Aripirazol prescription, (2) groups of Olanzapine prescription (including Aripirazol), and (3) groups of SSRIs prescription. Through these prescriptions, the effectiveness of Olanzapine was investigated and determined.

As these studies were retrospective investigations, and because they were performed by use of DSM-IV-TR, strange results and conclusions were expected.

	Aripirazol	**Olanzapine**	**SSRIs**	**Others**	**Total**
Total Cases	45	104=45	132*	125	453
	SSRIs*: Fluvoxamine(79%), Paroxetine(18%), Sertorarine(3%)				

Figure 4: The Relationship between number of subjects and the first prescriptions

Results

Histories of the prescriptions on each group

All histories of the prescriptions are shown in Figure 5, below, and were classified into five groups, as follows.

1. Olanzapine was prescribed, and according to its effect, the prescription was changed to Aripirazol. 54 cases were so switched, and they continued under this prescription.
2. Olanzapine was prescribed, and improvement occurred. Aripirazol was then added with the expectation of additional improvement, but, instead, the patients' situations deteriorated. Result: improvement was seen only after the Olanzapine prescription. 50 cases.
3. SSRI was prescribed as an antidepressant, according to DSM-IV-TR guidelines. No improvement was shown. Neither was improvement noted after the addition of other antidepressants. Afterwarad, Olanzapine was prescribed. Dramatic improvement was noted. 90 cases.
4. SSRI was prescribed as an antidepressant, according to DSM-IV-TR guidelines. No improvement was shown. Neither was improvement noted after the addition of other antidepressants. The prescription was then changed to only Aripirazol. No improvement was shown. Finallly, Olanzapine was prescribed and dramatic improvement was noted. 42 cases.
5. Olanzapine was prescribed to patients who had never before taken Olanzapine, in spite of psychopathological indication. Dramatic improvement was noted. 42 cases.

The dosage of Olanzapine was from 3mg to 20mg per day, which is officially permitted. As a result, any pathological change in the organs of the subjects was never observed through chemical or physical examinations.

There was no contamination with drugs that could introduce the complication of diabetes mellitus.

Other substances known to cause complication were excluded: hypertensive drugs, hyperlipemia drugs, laxatives. and vitamin B12.

Increase in body weight was observed in some cases, but as the disease improved, fat turned to muscle as a result of the patients' effort.

Olanzapine→Aripirazol: 54 cases
Olanzapine→Aripirazol+Olanzapine→Olanzapine: 50 cases
SSRIs→(More than 3 drugs) →Olanzapine: 90 cases
SSRIs→(More than 3 drugs) →Aripirazol→Olanzapine: 42 cases
Olanzapine: 42 cases

Figure 5: The Relationship between histories of prescriptions and number of patients

Differences between Single- and Multiple-Prescription Groups

The differences between the single-drug group and multiple-drug group are shown in Figure 6, below.

The number of clients who showed improvement on multiple drugs was overwhelmingly larger than the number of clients who showed improvement on a single drug. This phenomenon demonstrates the limitation of single-drug prescriptions. However, even though the effectiveness of the single-drug prescription approach has shown great limitation, this approach continues to be prevalent in the mainstream medical practice from the 1980s until today.

It is logical that the overall effectiveness of multiple-drug prescriptions is greater than the effectiveness of a single drug. Two drugs, for instance, can cover each other by reducing the possibility of harmful side effects. Another example: it has been commonly known that a prescription using one SSRI together with a Benzodiazepine derivative drug induces rapid improvement of anxiety and sleep disturbance As a result, it is almost inevitable that a prescription will broaden to include other drugs during the course of treatment for a disease or disorder. In this connection, a prescription of more than ten drugs was never rare, but, in fact, common.

Furthermore, psychosomatic diseases should be treated with a drug that targets the symptom, and also other drugs that affect the central nervous system as follows: antihypertensive drugs and SSRIs, including Benzodiazepine derivatives for essential hypertensions have been commonly prescribed to avoid sudden accidents and to reduce possibilities of side effects due to the mechanism of the disease.

Single drug prescription group	51
Multiple drug prescription group	392
TOTAL	443

Figure 6: Differences between the single- and multiple-prescription groups

Immunological Results

The effect of combined drugs on infections over three years was studied to determine how the immune system responded to antipsychotics.Figure 7, below.

Results showed that 18 cases of the Olanzapine single-prescription group and 297 cases of the multiple-prescriptions group experienced bacterial infective diseases. Zero case of the Olanzapine single-prescription group and 11 cases of multiple-prescription group experienced viral infections. Additionally, both CD3 (Tcell) and natural-killer cell activity elevated after prescription of Olanzapine on some, but not all, patients, compared with pre-prescription of Olanzapine

	Olanzapine	**Other Antipsychotics**
Bacterial Infections	n=18	n=297
Viral Infections	n=0	n=11
Additional results	(n=12)	(n=54)
NK Cell Activity	6.34+2.34	2.98+0.98
CD3 (mean, SD)	80.12+15.71	74.23+13.02
CD4 (mean, SD)	46.41+18.12	41.02+12.56
CD8 (mean, SD)	41.82+19.86	36.22+18.99

Figure 7: Immunological Results (related to some Infections)

Chapter IV: Improvement with Olanzapine

In this section, I will describe individual cases in which prescriptions were changed during the course of treatment, followed by some common questions and discussion.

Since these studies were performed by a retrospective investigation of all the patients, there were some strange additional prescriptions and changes of medications. It was consequently the obvious fact that these cases were Olanzapine effective.

All of these cases were diagnosed based on DSM-IV-TR, and all cases were subject to psychopathological follow-up examinations every month. When diagnoses based on DSM-IV-TR differed from psychopathological opinions, DSM-IV-TR took precedence. But when diseases and syndromes such as "the kernel schizophrenia" showed up in DSM-IV-TR, they were diagnosed by use of traditional psychopathological diagnostic criteria.

Indications of Olanzapine in the History of Prescriptions

Olanzapine > Aripirazol: 54 cases

This seems to be the most commonly performed method, called the "switching method." But diagnoses of patients at the first medical examination were classified as follows: 39 cases were schizoaffective disorders and 15 cases were schizophrenia.

Some typical cases are described below.

Case 1. 32-year- old female, an office worker in a large corporation

Character before illness: few friends, not so social but interested in music, sometimes went to musical concerts with her friends. Not so introverted, but giving a silent impression, sometimes losing awareness of immediate social context, always friendly with others.

History & Course of Illness: After graduating from the economics department of a private university; she entered employment as an office worker in a large corporation located near her home. After a three-month induction course, she was posted to the statistics department where she took statistics by use of a personal computer. She expected that her future would be atypical of a female employee who graduated university in economics. She always emphasized to others that she would never marry because she is happiest when she is working. Although she did not have an especially friendly association with others, she always accepted invitations to Karaoke and dinner, when she was invited by her superiors and fellow workers.

She took lunch with only one fellow worker or by herself because there were usually only two employees in her place of duty.

After three years of working for this corporation, she suddenly informed her superior that she wished to take one week's paid vacation, and she took a trip to Europe. Her superior was surprised to receive a sudden request for a holiday, but he concluded that this is common behavior among contemporary females. And so, he announced to the other workers that it was acceptable to make sudden vacation requests.

After she returned from her vacation, she worked at her usual duties in her work place. Since her work involved watching the screen of a personal computer, many of her fellow employees worked by reading aloud. For example, "Since to compare A group with B group, neglect the C group, and enter D, the answer will have to be X." In fact, this kind of monologue was always audible in her place of duty. So it was not unusual that she always talked to herself, even loudly sometimes, and asked of others, "Why were the results shown in such a strange format? I am sure that someone is trying to obstruct my work because the result must be X when this figure is entered. Who is interfering with me?" Although she suddenly began to declare who obstructed her work, her superior overlooked her behavior as nothing out of the ordinary. Her colleagues, also, did not bring her behavior into question.

Since her return from her trip to Europe, it gradually became difficult for her to submit the print-outs of her reports and receive the approval of her supervisor, so her supervisor gradually came to feel something strange in her behavior. Eventually, he asked her if something were wrong. She answered calmly, "Nothing, only my work is overdue." From then on, since it was difficult for her to submit her reports on time, she worked all night every day.

Her supervisor understood that it is against the law to require a female employee to work through the night, and that her habit of working all night became his responsibility. He suggested to her in a kind voice that she is not required to work all night; he further suggested that she could postpone her unfinished work until the following week. But she immediately responded, "I have just understood that all my fellow workers, including you, are trying to obstruct my work by saying such a thing! You, along with all the members of this company, have always been obstructing my work! I have been trapped!"

Her superior was shocked at her response, but asked her kindly, "Are you troubled by anything? If so, let me know about it." She answered in restrained anger, "You, the chief, already understood what was going on. I would like to request that you stop torturing me!"

The supervisor tried to reason with her. He invited her to speak about anything that might be bothering her; he asked if any of her colleagues were interfering with her; he even offered to reduce her workload. But she angrily rejected all his offers. Finally, she accused him of being responsible for the "torment and bullying" she was experiencing.

The supervisor was confused by her attitude; he thought she was suffering from exhaustion, and he realized that the matter needed more professional attention than he could offer. He directed her to visit the company's doctor on the very next day.

The doctor asked her a number of questions to try to determine what could be the cause of this young woman's difficulties at work, but she refused to respond to his questions and remained silent for the half-hour interview. The doctor reported to her supervisor that she should be examined by a psychiatric specialist, and he wrote a letter of introduction.

The letter of introduction that I received from this doctor suggested that the young woman was seriously depressed and was possibly suicidal.

Shortly afterward, this woman suddenly appeared in my clinic without an appointment. Nevertheless, I decided to examine her immediately. As soon as she entered my room, she suddenly began to cry loudly and continued for some time, as if she had finally reached at safe place. I accepted this situation and allowed her to cry for nearly an hour. Then, cautiously, I asked her if she would let me help her, and she immediately answered, "Help me, but I do not want to talk about details." I let her know that I understood and that I would like to help her as soon as possible, but I suggested that the first step would be a rest for several weeks, and I asked her if she would agaree to take some medication that would help to give her brain a rest. And she agreed.

I prescribed a low dosage (a 5mg tablet) of Olanzapine once a day for two weeks, and she agreed to receive regular medical treatment as an outpatient under the diagnosis of schizoaffective disorder.

The next day, just as I expected, she called to complain that she could not sleep, and I asked her to increase her dosage of Olanzapine to two tablets per day. She complied, and she was able to sleep. And she showed up for her weekly sessions.

During her sessions, she began to complain about what happened in her company. She said that she had been treated harshly in the past. All her experiences were described in the past tense, even though the situation was actually ongoing. "I cannot recognize the situation in terms of plain facts," she told me. And then the subject of her complaints changed to her mood and activity from bad experiences in the past. She frequently said, "Although I will have to return to my work, I have no confidence about doing my work." And she asked me to prescribe some medicine to make her cheer up. So I prescribed Aripirazol (6mg/day).

At her next visit, I was surprised to hear her complaint that, in spite of increased energy, she had also become restless. I asked her to reduce by half her dose of Aripirazol, and two weeks later when she visited my office, she seemed like a healthy girl. She told me that she wanted to return to work since she was bored with trying to find ways to kill time.

I saw that this young woman was in remission, so I wrote the official diagnostic letter for her, saying that she is in remission, and that she can return to work.

When she was examined by the company's doctor, however, he noticed that her wrist bandaged and he assumed, without further investigation, that the patient had attempted suicide, and he sent me a letter declaring that the patient had tried to commit suicide and that she would have to receive more treatment and more rest and that she would not be permitted to return to work. He asked me to write a letter confirming his analysis and ordering the necessity of more rest for this patient and prohibiting her from returning to work.

I was surprised to read this letter because I had already confirmed that the wrist injury was due to a fall down a craggy slope at the seashore. When I actually examined and treated this injury, I could see that it was not caused by a wrist cut. I informed the company doctor of this fact and included my medical findings. But, the company doctor sent a letter saying that he had already prohibited the patient's return to work due to a suicidal scar and that if I refused to write a letter confirming this analysis, the patient would be dismissed from her position with the company due to an absence without due medical confirmation. So I had no choice but to write the medical letter suggesting a rest for one year.

After this, the young woman came to my clinic on the verge of tears about this situation. She continued to receive psychotherapy once a month, and she continued taking 5ms of Olanzapine and 3mg of Aripirazol every day. She asserted that she would not experience a relapse. She got a job at a fast-food restaurant, which she kept of one year.

One day, she visited me to tell me that she had received official permission to return to work from another company doctor, since the regular doctor was transferred to another area. Her personality seemed active and cheerful, by contrast to her demeanor of the previous year.

Back at work, her supervisor assigned her to new department to give her a fresh start, and she did well. She continued taking 3mg of Aripirazol, but it is not clear whether Aripirazol is responsible for preventing her relapse.

Short discussion: When this young woman was diagnosed according to DSM-IV-TR guidelines, she was given a diagnosis of schizophrenia by many specialists. But it would be difficult to diagnose her as schizophrenic based on her personality before the illness because her pre-illness personality differed from the typical schizophrenic personality. From another point of view, she might be suitably diagnosed with a typical psychosis.

When medications were considered for her, her persistent silence and unresponsive behavior were considered. She might be suffering from a disturbance of consciousness. Furthermore, her pathological experiences, such as delusional ideation and auditory hallucinations, subsided within several days after beginning to take Olanzapine.

It is a contemporary trend among those who have experience in higher education to be unsociable, sometimes to have not even one close friend. So this young woman's personality could be simply contemporary, not schizophrenic. However, it should be noted that she became friendly toward me and toward her psychologist after knowing us for less than a month.

Since I never found evidence of any pathologic experience like a hallucination and delusion in this young woman for one year, she could be appropriately diagnosed as having schizoaffective disorder.

She could also be diagnosed with schizophrenia by psychiatrists based on symptomatic evidence, and consequently, she could be told that she would have no possibility of ever returning to work.

It was not clarified whether 3mg of Aripirazol prevented her relapse, and, if so, to what extent or degree. Alternatively, if 3mg of Aripirazol contributed to her relapse, was the dosage enough to prevent such a relapse? Prospective observation will have to be performed on her in the future.

Case 2. a 24-year-old male, technician in a large company

Personality before illness: introverted, gentle, no friends, unsociable, and precision, round trip between company and dormitory.

Course of illness and treatment: After a graduation from a local high school, he found work in a small company but he quit this work after two years due to trouble with his fellow workers. He told his parents that he wanted to work in a large company, and he did find work in a big company that was located at the outskirts of a large town. After his introductory course, he was assigned to as an engineer trainee. At first, he worked quietly and when he did not understand something, he asked his superior politely and listened to his superior's suggestions. He willingly worked overtime hours, and he was recognized as a model employee.

But one day, he suddenly became excited and he shouted that the supervisor is always watching him and infringing his privacy. And he began to destroy the surveillance cameras. "You are always manipulating me through a laser beam," he shouted. And he continued to shout that he would put an end to this behavior."You shall die," he cried as he began to destroy machines that were in his path.

Other employees who witnessed this scene were astonished because this behavior seemed so out of character, but they seen were able to subdue him and carry him to the company doctor, who—after receiving the appropriate authorizations—brought the man to my clinic.

When he entered into the clinic, he calmed down and quietly waited for his examination.

Course of treatments from the first examination: Although the patient entered into the examination room quietly, once inside, he began to complain angrily, "Doctor! All of them have always tried to manipulate me through a laser beam, and they keep watch on me by setting cameras everywhere!" And he implored, "Doctor! Set me free!"

Although the patient was restricted by his fellows, I felt there was a possibility of sudden violent behavior, so I spoke very quietly to the man and told him that I could see what kind of predicament he was in, and I could see that he was very tired. I told him that if he would agree, I would like to give him a tablet that would let him rest. He said he believed me and he would accept the table. "But," he added, "If I find out that you are a part of this gang, I will kill you."

I gave the patient a 5mg tablet of Olanzapine-zydis, and the patient asked in sleepy voice, "May I take a sleep? I have not slept in over a week." But by then, he had already fallen into a deep sleep and was snoring loudly. His fellows, who had just witnessed his violent behavior, asked if they should take the man to the hospital and check him in. They were worried what his behavior would be when he woke up. But I told them that the man's rapid response to the Olanzapine was a good sign, and that if he sleeps until the next morning or noon, everything will be fine and his behavior will return to normal. Even if he seems to be irritable, he will still show presence of mind.

They took turns keep watch over the patient until the next morning and keep the supervisors apprised of his situation, according to the supervisors' request. It was well that they accepted their superior's order; if they had admitted him to the hospital, he would have had to pay a lot of money.

The patient slept uninterrupted until noon of the next day. When he awakened he was surprised to see his surroundings and to note that a number of senior people from his company were present. "What happened?" he asked. One of the supervisors asked him, "Don't you remember anything? Have you no remembrance of what you did and what you complained about?"

The patient answered, "Did I do something wrong? Did I make trouble? Please tell me why many supervisors are here."

One of the supervisors began speaking to the patient as if to a very offensive person, asking him "What? You don't you know what you did?" But quickly, another of the supervisors quieted this fellow, reminding him that I had told them never to make the patient remember the last day's events. So the excited speaker changed his tone and said, "You didn't do anything wrong; you suddenly lost consciousness and fell down. And so, we carried you to the doctor and kept watching you until you recovered consciousness."

But the patient seemed doubtful. "It seems strange that so many of supervisors came to stay here with me," he said, and he asked why he had lost consciousess and what kind of fall he experienced because he felt serious pain in all of his muscles.

"Trust the doctor," one of supervisors suggesting gently.

The patient agreed to this idea, then he fell once again into a deep sleep. Seeing this man sleeping peacefully, no one was able to believe that just a day earlier, he had destroyed a number of machines in his work place.

The patient stayed at the clinic and I gave him an intravenous drip injection, because, he had not had anything to drink or eat for more than twelve hours.

Since the medication was still effective after half a day or more, and even with such a low dosage, I knew that the patient would not become excited or display this inappropriate, destructive behavior again. I prescribed the same medicine for continuation. And I requested authorization from the supervisors for the patient to visit the clinic again by himself. I was sure he would improve and recover very soon.

The next day, he visited the clinic for his examination by himself, though he was somewhat dazed from the experience. As soon as he entered the examination room, he asked to be told what had happened and what he had done, but I simply told him that he had been seriously tired—mentally exhausted, even, due to serious sleep disturbance. I told him that he should not worry about what happened because his condition improved by only one tablet of medicine, but if he does experience the same disturbance, he should visit me immediately.

Then he explained to me that it had became so difficult for him to sleep at night, that he had tried a number of sleeping pills, but nothing had worked and it had been a long time since he had been able to sleep at all. And at some point, he lost consciousness and couldn't remember anything until he woke up in my office and he could not figure out what had gone on or where he was or why. And at that point, he still felt lethargic and exhausted mood and in a depressive mood. He asked me if I could prescribe something to help.

I willingly prescribed a tablet of 3mg of Aripirazol 3mg and asked him to try this for two weeks at first. Afterward, the patient continued on this drug and after some time, his condition improved completely.

However, because the incident in his workplace was officially judged as destructive behavior by this employer, he had to leave the company, and he had to leave his room in the dormitory. As a result, he had to find an apartment and some new work. He went to a public employment security office every day and he managed to live on his a severance allowance in the meantime. After a month, he found new work. At the time, he was judged completely recovered, and he did not need to continue with visits to the clinic. From then on—for more than three years at the last check-in—he was employed at that same company, and has been promoted to the head of is work area, and he has experienced no relapses.

Short discussion on this case: The patient was diagnosed with a typical schizoaffective disorder, showing sudden onset, and symptomatically unremarkable pathological experiences like hallucination and delusion due to disturbance of consciousness. There was no remarkable character trait and the patient was socially adapted. It is well known that Olanzapine zydis tablets show remarkable results for these kinds of symptoms, empirically and psycho-pharmacologically. This profile is consistent with the definition of Pauleikhoff, B. and Hatotani, T. (2)(3), and is thought to be responsive to immediate diagnosis and treatment. An element of this profile is a tendency to repeat, and consequently a long-term prescription is warranted to prevent relapse.

It is not rare that similar cases that come to immediate remission only by 5mg of Olanzapine zydis tablets. In other words, the fundamental formula of Rest→Recovery of Integration→Improvement of Depression, was shown.

Only a short term depressive state was observed in this case, but it is possible that any difficulty in recovery of the depressive state was caused by the Aripirazol. In other words, it is doubtful that the depressive state in this case was improved by the so-called "switching method."

In any event, although this case was never diagnosed as schizophrenia, it could be said that Olanzapine was extremely effective in managing, if not curing, it.

None of the 54 cases in this study showed praecox feelings, and none showed unnatural Aida (interval), which was argued by Kimura, B.

Unexpected sudden and unusual behaviors—for example, the matter of the young woman in Case 1., above—have been thought to be psychopathological behavior that emerges just before the onset of schizophrenia. But, as far as we can see from the course of remission, such as behavior could be considered a common feature of contemporary people(12)-(20). Even if her unexpected European trip were the special behavior associated with pre-onset of schizophrenia, her symptoms, psychopathologically, should have continued for a long time, even until nearly the end of her life. But, on the contrary, she actually improved and went into remission within a short time. So it is very difficult to give her a diagnosis of schizophrenia.

Despite the discoveries in this case, this young woman would be diagnosed with schizophrenic disorder according to DSM-IV-TR guidelines.

In the last analysis, it has been shown that symptomatic classifications or diagnoses like DSM-IV-TR are never based on scientific anthropology but are only superficial classifications.

Olanzapine > Aripirazol+Olanzapine > Olanzapine : 50 Cases

These prescription methods are considered the most common. But, since normal methods are not always common, I will describe some typical cases, below:

Case. A 33-year-old female, housewife and part-timer worker

Personality before illness: relatively social; usually went shopping with her friends; not a meticulous personality; seemed to be a typical contemporary woman.

History of illness and treatment: After graduating from a local private university in English Literature, she found work in a financial institution that was in the same town as her university. She entered this workplace with a fanfare. She was devoted to her work and she worked well with the company's clients. She had no problems during her working time. However, she felt free to take breaks during the day, even when other staff members were working and doing business. Such behavior was usually observed in local financial institutions these days, and no one reprimanded her for it. Only the most senior employees were irritated by it. But they, too, said nothing, since they understood it seemed to be the custom among some of the younger employees. In addition, they feared to mention the problem to the employee, lest she went immediately to the Labor Standards Inspection Office to report sexual harassment or power-harassment. But the senior employees continued to grumbled about the situation.

The young woman in our study had entered this financial institution, primarily, to find a clever and suitable husband among the other employees, but when she saw that all the male employees were dull and accepting of unreasonable demands from their superiors, she changed her mind about marrying any of her colleagues. Finally, however, when she was 26, she did marry a man who worked in the higher echelons of the company. A big wedding reception was held and her branch manager was invited. She continued working after the wedding because she wished to have the luxury of two incomes.

When this woman was 27, she became pregnant, and she delivered a healthy baby. And so, she seemed to be very happy, but as her baby grew, she began to feel inconvenienced by the child's presence in her life. She decided to deposit her baby in a nursery school so she could have more free time, but even so, she felt unbearably restrained, especially when she became pregnant with a second baby. She felt that she had to have more time to herself. Even though she did have free time, it was difficult for her to go out during the pregnancy, and she complained repeatedly, "Set me free, and set me free."

Her husband was an able employee, and he was the prodigy of the big boss in a large trading company. As a result, he worked very hard, and he often returned home as late as midnight. His wife had never experienced or witnessed such long working hours in a financial institution, and she did not believe that he was actually working all that time, and she began to doubt him. She noticed that he was not interested in sex with her because he was exhausted, he said.

She began to wait up for her husband to arrive home so she could assess the smell and appearance of his clothing. She was convinced he was having an affair and she decided that she would catch him in the act. Soon, her suspicions began to show in her behavior. As soon as her husband left home for work, she immediately went to her parents' home to leave her children in their care, and she kept constant watch on her husband, even loitering in front of the company's building. Sometimes, she returned home after him, when he finished his work and returned home earlier than usual. But, on such occasions, she questioned her husband with sharp eyes and demanded to know why he returned home earlier than usual. "Did some trouble happen between someone and you?" she would ask, sarcastically. Even on holidays, when sometimes the husband had to work, she had even more severe words for him.

As time passed, the woman said she heard some female voice through her husband's cell phone even when they were at home together. The voices said things like: "Can you meet me today?" or "I am desperate to see you today." Furthermore, when she was playing with her children at home, she heard female voices saying, "He has already left you because you have been too selfish to live together with him," and sometimes, "Since he loves only me and he is mine, you must leave his house."

Such voices seemed truly audible to the woman, and she came to firmly believe that her husband and a lover were already trying to throw her out. As these voices increased, she blamed her husband more and more. But he did not understand what was happening to her and he was at a loss.

She started following him all day because of the strange voices she was hearing and because of her doubts about his fidelity to her. He felt that her behavior was too strange and, at last, he decided to find out what happened to her and why she was not herself, but appeared to be someone else, instead.

He began to investigate her behavior. After he went work every morning, he quietly returned home to observe her behavior. He was shocked to see what she was doing, and consequently, he understood the meaning of her strange behavior.

He tried to explain to his wife what was really going on in his life, but he realized that she heard only a hallucinative voice saying, "No! No! Your husband is giving a false story. He is trying to trick you into believing his lies." She became angry and excitable, and she started crying, but she did not seem confused.

Her husband suggested that she begin to see a psychiatrist, but she immediately responded to him that he's the one who should visit a psychiatrist. He urged her again and again, but she emphatically rejected this proposal every time. Finally, the young husband came to me with this problem, and I suggested that he come to visit me and bring his wife along. So the husband told his wife that he had decided to see a psychiatrist, and he wanted her to accompany him.

When we sat together in my office, I told them that I could see they were exhausted with each other, and I suggested that they take a rest and I told them I would like to prescribe some medicines for both of them. Additionally, I told them, you should both receive family counseling. I prescribed a placebo for the husband and Olanzapine for his wife.

The following day, the wife called me to say that she could not sleep for more than three hours and asked for additional medicine, so I suggested taking two Olanzapine 5mg tablets. Afterwards, the wife slept well, while her husband slept as before.

The husband decided to take a rest from his work and, with the help of the medical letter I wrote for him, he was permitted to take a vacation for several weeks. As time passed, the young wife's delusional ideas about her husband and her auditory hallucinations gradually subsided within a relatively short interval. However, while her pathological condition was improving, she complained of a reduction in activity and a depressive mood. I switched her prescription from Olanzapine to Aripirazol (Aripirazol 6mg), but no remarkable change was observed. Then I reduced the dosage of Olanzapine to 5mg and raised the dosage of Aripirazol to 12mg. Unfortunately, she became rather worse, complaining of severe sleep disturbance and serious depression, so I raised the Olanzapine to 10mg and discontinued the Aripirazol. After a month, both her sleep disturbance and depressive mood improved to the point of remission. And at last, after five months from the first visit, she was in complete remission. Her life is going smoothly. She and her husband returned to their original loving, supportive relationship, and they enjoy their home life with their children.

Nevertheless, the young wife continues monthly visits to me, but no pathologic finding has been found during the past two years.

Short discussion of this case: Before the widespread use of DSM-III, this case might have been diagnosed as the so-called typical "first period of the thirty-year-old delusional syndrome." Unfortunately, such a diagnostic disorder is little employed today. Now, it would be common for this patient to be diagnosed as schizophrenic according to DSM-IV-TR. This is a typical case that expresses differences between a psychopathological diagnosis and a superficial symptomatic diagnosis.

If I were to discuss this case psychopathologically or phenomenolgically, a conclusion could be as follows: as soon as this young woman completed the biggest event of her life (delivering a baby, and then another baby), her life was suddenly and dramatically changed. She had to rear two children without a break, and, of course, she had to manage their rebellious periods.

When the two children entered nursing school, she might have been able to relax. Unfortunately, however, just when she was able to have some relaxed time, her husband was under constant strain from his work. Consequently, although her life style changed from extreme strain to a more relaxed situation, her husband was not available to interact with her or to be present for her, so she reacted defensively. In other words, when she was freed from an exhausting situation, she was still not able to take a rest. In such a blocked situation, it is not unexpected that she could fall into a mental framework of breakup and collapse. I suspect that her collapse took the form of a delusion of jealousy.

This case represents an appropriate Olanzapine target situation. Olanzapine produces a healing effect in cases of exhaustion. On exhaustion, Olanzapine works as activating agent, i.e., at first, it works on the Dopamin, which is a naturally occurring agent in the brain that addresses exhaustion. And, as the situation improves, the Olanzapine works to assist Serotonin. Some practitioners insist that Aripirazol is the appropriate activating agent in an exhaustion case such as this, but in my judgment and experience, it invites only a worse effect, since Aripirazol is a stimulant. In fact, it was shown in this case that Aripirazol did not work.

This case clearly shows that only Olanzapine worked sufficiently to induce healing activity from exhaustion. Thus, this case must be diagnosed as a paranoid syndrome, described by Zutt, J., instead of schizoprenia. Olanzapine was the most effective agent to this situation (27).

SSRIs > Numerous Prescriptions > Olanzapine : 90 Cases

Case. 46-year-old male, department head in a middle-class company

Character before illness: earnest, precise, social, obliging, no special hobby, but interested in a many subjects.

Course of illness and treatment: While he was growing up, he became gradually aware of mood fluctuations. In his words: "I had already noticed my mood ups and downs from adolescence. When I was in a high mood, I thought I could do everything so I took on many projects. But as soon as I completed the largest task, I fell into melancholy. Once when I got depressed, I remained in a depressive mood. I could not stop taking time off from my University studies. This went on for a long time; consequently, I had to repeat a year in University two times."

Although his advisors and fellows regarded him as a manic-depressive, they did not suggest that he get a medical examination by a psychiatric specialist; he was absent for only two days of preparation for the comprehensive graduation exams.

It was not necessary for him to repeat a year in University, certainly not two years. Many students who missed only two days of comp. prep. Continued without repeating at all. But this young man had always boasted that we he would graduate in the top level of his class. Therefore, he took it upon himself to repeat two years of university.

After graduation, he wished to continue to graduate school, but he was not sure what he wanted to study and he was not accepted into any post-graduate program. So, instead of graduate school, he found a position as an executive trainee in a company that manufactured precision machinery, since his uncle was the president of the company.

He worked long hours and he worked very hard, including work of a more senior employee. Sometimes he was still at his work until midnight. His fellow employees started asking him when he sleeps. He received good evaluations and he achieved good results for the company, so of course he was promoted to the head of a department by the time he was 30, and by the time he was 40, he was promoted again.

During that time, he took as much as a week of continuous holidays, due to his difficulty in getting up in the morning, but no superior complained of his behavior because of the extra work that he did.

As a senior employee, he took care of his subordinates, even after his promotions, so he was always liked and respected by them. Unfortunately, during a serious economic downturn, the amount of his own work increased, but the work and duties of his subordinate decreasing; therefore, the overall quality of the work of the department decreased.

His work was, at first, to begin the review of future plans, and the reclamation of new plans and new customers to improve their markets. This was very big work and he had to work all night, sometimes even for days.

The president of the company, seeing him working so long and hard, suggested that he should cut a few corners in his work in order to stay healthy. He took this suggestion, but it suddenly transpired that he could not get to sleep easily at night and he could not get up in the morning. At that point, he began to think that he must complete one project right after the next, nevermind how late it was or how hard he was working. And this soon became a way of life for him.

However, one day he suddenly snapped and he started shouting, "The whole world is suddenly falling to pieces and it is making an unbelievably loud noise!" "It is the end of the world!" "There is no hope!" After that, he seemed always to be talking to himself, and did not respond to other people's questions or remarks. And, at last, the man, accompanied with his fellows, visited my clinic.

During out first session, he began to describe his situation in a calm voice, as a normal person would do. He explained that he has recently found it difficult to concentrate on his work, though he must complete a number of projects. He feels his energy for his work diminishing. And, he said, he is in a seriously depressive frame of mind and sometimes just can't do his work. "I felt I must disappear," he told me.

During this session, he did not express any pathologic behavior or speech, like claiming imminent world destruction. He made himself appear to be in a normal mental state; he behaved as if there was no disturbance of his consciousness. I diagnosed him as having major depression, based on DSM-IV-TR. But, of course, I had already intuited his his disturbance of consciousness. I wanted to prescribe Olanzapine, but, the patient refused. He told me that he thinks he is suffering from depression, and he said that Olanzapine would not be effective for him because he knows that Olanzapine is usually prescribed for schizophrenia. He specifically requested one of the SSRIs or some antidepressants.

It can't be helped that Fluvoxamine 50mg, Flutoprazepam 2mg and Lormetazepam 10mg were commonly prescribed for depression, along with continuing psychotherapy, so I decided to make this prescription, as the patient had requested, and wait until he complained of no improvement of the depression, but changing instead to the manic stated as an effect of the Fluvoxamine.

Even if this patient had experienced atypical psychotic symptoms, called schizoaffective disorder, I thought the possibility of his relapse would be minimal.

When he came for his second visit the following week, he complained that although he had slept well and for a longer time, and while he wish to return to work, he actually has no motivation to work. I explained that we should wait to see what effect the medication will have, then make a course of treatment. After a month, the man had gradually requested other antidepressant or additional medicines, since he did not improve on the original prescription (as I had expected). So I changed his prescription of Paroxetine from 10mg to 40mg for four months. I decided to accept his requests because I knew that he did not take any medicines except the requested medicines. His next request was Fluvoxamine 100mg and Paroxetine 20mg. After this, he began to suffer from serious sleep disturbance and even the possibility of relapse into schizoaffective disorder.

The time had come for me to urge this patient to switch from his current prescriptions to the medicine that I originally suggested: Olanzapine. The man did not refuse my suggestion because, for one thing, he was in a condition of clouded consciousness. So he began to take a 5mg tablet of Olanzapine 5mg. He complained that at the night he could not sleep for more than three hours, so I increased his prescription of Olanzapine to 10mg. From this, he gradually improved, and within several weeks, his complaint subsided. Instead, he began to assert that he is now strong and vigorous and he wanted to return to work. Though I expected the patient to improve, I was surprised to see how suddenly he improved.

He returned to his full emotional personality and he was able to communicate well. Still, I suggested that he continue to rest from his work for a few more months, worrying that he might lapse into the manic state. But my fears were not realized; he continued to lead a normal life.

Some problems did remain, however. The patient was able to recover from his depressive-manic disorder by a prescription of Olanzapine, which is officially prescribed for schizophrenia. Although I tried repeatedly to diagnose him as schizophrenia by using the DSM-IV-TR, I could not find schizophrenic symptoms in his course of illness.

When the patient did return to work, I strongly advised him to take it easy and to not take on a full work load at first. As soon as he returned his work, however, he found a lot of work waiting for him and he saw that it would be difficult to do reduce his workload and, in any case, the idea of starting slow and gradually increasing his work-time was not permitted in his department, even though I sent a letter recommending a reduced workload until the patient re-acclimated himself to his work place. So he could not help working hard and completing more than a full day's work within a few hours. In fact, once, when the president of the company went abroad for an extended trip, the patient is the one who performed the work of the absent president.

From then on, when the patient's dosage of Olanzapine was reduced (down to 5mg), he experienced exhaustion in appearance and performance, so the dosage has been maintained at 10mg with excellent results.

Today, the patient's uncle has retired from the presidency of the company and has become chairman of the board, instead. The current president of the company is none other than the patient under discussion in this case. He is still taking 10mg of Olanzapine and he says that this medicine saved his life. "I would have to leave the presidency of the company if Olanzapine did not exist," he says.

Short discussion of the case: This patient showed extraordinary improvement with Olanzapine. If I had heard of his behavior in his workplace before he began treatment with Olanzapine, I may well have recognized only a biological reaction and diagnosed his disorder as atypical psychosis or schizoaffective disorder. I may even have recommended immediate admission to a psychiatric hospital.

We could speculate that nearly all of the patient's A10-nerve work areas were working independently and, consequently, his brain may have been cerebropathologically falling into an integrative disturbance situation. We might also speculate that all of the brain, midbrain, amygdaloid nucleus (related to emotion, fear, adaptability), hippocampus, basal ganglia (related to somatic motor), nucleus accumbens (related to limbic system, known as the emotional and visceral brain) and frontal association area (related to personality, movement motivation and planning), works independently. Since such situations are thought to exist only in biological areas, they are commonly treated only by medication.

In the current case, although the patient had come through some serious experiences, he behaved gently, as if in a normal depression, not as though he had experienced anything especially dramatic. I considered him a very rare personality.

Although he was at first diagnosed with major depression, he never showed any response or improvement with any antidepressants or a combination of antidepressants. He responded only to Olanzapine. And as his exhaustion improved with Olanzapine, his illness seemed also to improve.

However, the deeper question could be whether he suffers from a core schizophrenia, because of his lack of human relationships with other people and his tendency to be out of sync others. It is commonly expected that a high-intelligent core schizophrenics will break down into psychopathology at some point in their lives.

When this patient was diagnosed as a non symptomatic core schizophrenic, it was expected that he would experience remission due to the selective effect of Olanzapine on the A10 nerves. (Unfortunately, non-symptomatic schizophrenia is considered a "negative symptom of schizophrenia" in the symptomatic diagnostic manuals.)

Thus, we speculate, this patient was able to retain his natural ability to adjust to life's events because of his high intelligence and Olanzapine. In this connection, this speculation is in agreement with theories about the relationship between brain and spirit, as outlined and argued by Penfield, W.

With the current case, some diagnostic problems remain. The patient was able to recover with the help of Olanzapine, which is officially prescribed only for schizophrenia. Although I tried repeatedly to diagnose him as schizophrenic according to DSM-IV-TR, I could not find schizophrenic symptoms in his course of illness.

In any event, this case would not be diagnosed as schizophrenia based on the symptomatic classification manual, but by the Olanzapine-effective situation based on the suitable psychopathological consideration. Additionally, this case could ordinarily be diagnosed as major depression, but to satisfy the requirements of this diagnosis, the patient would have to be actually in a deep pathogenetic situation. Such cases are commonly observed in standard clinical examinations. Thus, it is understood that when patients are diagnosed as in a depressive state, their pathogeneses were unexpectedly deep.

SSRIs > (Numerous prescriptions) > Aripirazol > Olanzapine: 42 cases

These categories of disease are diagnosed as major depressions, on which SSRIs are extremely effective, according to the symptomatic classification manual, DSM-IV-TR, and they are similar to the types of cases described earlier. But, according to these actual experiences, Olanzapine was shown to improve these cases under a psychopathogenetic diagnosis, and the patients' condition became worse with Aripirazol, although it has been argued that Aripirazol is effective not only as an activating agent, but also to treat borderline personality disorders. However, as I learned directly from Prof. Casey at the University of Oregon, this medicine has been shown to worsen patients' conditions, while Olanzapine was shown to cause improvement.

I wish to present typical evidence, as shown in the following case, which is simply expressed, though nearly all cases are similar.

Case. 33-year-old male, independent businessman

Personality before illness: enthusiasm for his work, precise, avoided quarrels, well-mannered. Hobby: the art of flower arranging.

History of illness and treatment: He was raised indulgently. His father was adopted by his mother's family and given absolute authority over the family, consistent with local tradition. His father has long been accorded special treatment from his mother's parents. In the whole extended family, there was never any opposition to his father.

However, within this framework, whatever he wanted, even if it was too expensive for a child, he could get it immediately. So he grew up in the blind love of his parents and grandparents. And all his father's hope rested on his shoulders.

Unfortunately, as he grew older, his father was ashamed of him because of his unmasculine behavior and ideations. And so it happened that his father was resigned to his personality, while his mother doted on him for fear of her patents. In other words, he grew up in complex family.

Once day, when he was a young man, he suddenly announced to all his family members that he thought even an independent business man should have a university degree in order to continue the business. The family was surprised and expressed opposition to this idea. But, in spite of the opposition, he left home and entered law school, not the school of economics or business.

His family was very unhappy about this, since—they felt—law is the enemy of the independent business man. This was the first time he lost his temper with his parents and other members of his family, and he decided to conduct his life by himself.

As soon as he entered the university, he began to spend time with a different set of companions. And, unexpectedly, he neglected his school life and began to spend time in a mah-jongg parlor, where he was recognized as an outstanding player, and the owners of the parlor always asked him to stay around to attract customers to the parlor. So he fell into the habit of spending much of his time at mah-jongg and evidence of a gambling addiction began to surface.

He went to the university only for important occasions such as the promotion exams, although he never attended classes. At last, however, he did graduate with good results.

After graduation, he entered a training internship at an independent business, which lasted for about three years. He had no difficulty in this training period. He developed good relationships with the customers, and he was encouraged by many of them in his endeavors. They told him he should be his father's successor, and that he would be better than his father because his father is always drunk.

In fact, he did not wish to work with his father because his father was drinking all during the day. Furthermore, when his father always disappeared from the work whenever someone had to take responsibility for something, so our patient had to assume the responsibility of his father.

He began to remember that his biggest motivation to enter the university was to get away from home. Furthermore, when he entered university, he already decided to find some other kind of work that would relieve him of having to enter the family business. (Of course, he did not really wish to be a lawyer, since it was too difficult to be the lawyer in his university. He simply wished just to leave his home.)

Unfortunately, he had to live in his home, though it was strange for him—much worse than before he went away to school, since he had become used to living on his own. Nevertheless, he made the effort to receive his father's training and to succeed his father as the owner of his family business.

By the time he was 30, his father had retired from the business completely, and our patient, who had succeeded his family, both in name and in reality, began to reorganize the family business in terms of working methods and other good business practices.

Unfortunately, his father (though he was often drunk) continued to interfere in the running of the business because he objected to his son's abandoning the traditional style of doing business. Father and son often quarreled, but soon enough, the father saw that his son won every argument of logic and he realized it was useless for him to object, and he eventually went along with his son's ideas and methods.

The son worked harder and harder under his new business model. He worked long hours and even on holidays. He claimed to his customers that he would achieve results that were twice as impressive as his father's.

It was about this time that the young man's neighbors and fellows began to notice that his personality, even his character seemed to be undergoing some kind of change. He started to keep a low profile and to keep a smile on his face, though neither of these traits had been part of his makeup. But who could argue, because his business results increased until they doubled his father's, and this took him only three years.

Every day, he experienced dizziness; he would break into a cold sweat, and had difficulty standing up. He thought the situation might be caused by the insomnia he had been suffering for quite a long time, so he tried to sleep in bed, but he was only dazed. He could not sleep. He figured that if he did not feel sleepy and could not sleep, he may as well return to work. But, at this point, he could not even move. He couldn't understand what was happening and he was worried. He decided he should receive a drip injection of vitamins and nutrients, but he felt no change after the drip injection, so he went to the clinic, where the attending doctor suggested that he should visit a doctor of psychosomatic medicine or psychiatry, and the doctor referred this patient to my clinic.

In the first examination, he appeared to be seriously exhausted. He showed 75 points on the Self-Rating Depression Scale (SDS) by Zung, which was extremely high.

He asserted that he was suffering from depression, and from exhaustion. For the three years since he took over the family business from his father, he told me, he could not remember taking any rest. And, furthermore, there are all kinds of pressures associated with the work. And again, he told me that he is depressed. Because of the continuous complaints about depression, I began to suspect his story.

Nevertheless, he was diagnosed with major depression according to DSM-IV-TR, and Fluvoxamine 50mg a day was prescribed. After one month, he showed no improvement, so the prescription was increased to 100mg a day. After another month, there was, again, no improvement, so the prescription was switched to Paroxetine 40mg; then switched to Sertoraline 200mg. Then he was changed to Milnaciprane 100mg at his request. But, after three months, he still complained of the same symptoms. At last, the prescription was changed to three different kinds of upper-limit SSRIs, but his condition and complaints did not change.

Thus, when I reviewed his diagnosis history, I found his pathogenesis from the psychopathological point of view as follows: this young man had passed his life in a deeply pathological situation, and he came to exhibit symptoms of a borderline personality disorder. I began to prescribe Aripirazol 6mg, at the suggestion of Prof. Cassy. Then I gradually elevated the dosage of Aripirazol to 18mg over four months. But the young man's condition did not improve; it became worse. As a result, I decided to do a deeper investigation into his life history, from his birth until now, in order to try to discover what was at the basis of his unfortunate situation.

What I found was fundamental pathogenesis that included many difficulties and conflicts in his family situation. He shared the profile of the "defeat of a runaway," which means the onset of schizophrenia and the unnatural activity of the A10 nerves.

I immediately prescribed Olanzapine 5mg. After a waiting period, he complained that he still couldn't sleep for more than five hours every night, but that he does feel better. So, I raised the dose of Olanzapine to 10mg. His condition improved, and he requested a 28-day prescription. I assessed his condition as stable, and I knew he would not take the whole prescription at once, so I agreed to the 28-days prescription of Olanzapine.

After a month, the patient visited me at my clinic, but the interval between visits became longer and longer. He was given appointments for every month, but he often showed up for his appointments only every two or three months.

After four years (from the first prescription of Olanzapine 10mg) the patient continued to visit me to renew his 28-day prescription of Olanzapine. During these visits, we talk about his daily life and how he is managing. He tells me that he is healthy, but he is in a business slump, and he has headaches. He continues to miss any appointments that are not necessary for the purpose of renewing his prescription.

Short discussion of this case: Initially, because this patient seemed to have a melancholia-affinitive personality, and according to DSM-IV-TR, he was diagnosed as having major depression. But, I discovered a typical borderline-personality-disorder family situation when I reviewed the psychopathology of the case. At that point, I suspected that Olanzapine was the appropriate treatment for this patient. Unfortunately, diagnoses based on psychopathology have commonly not been permitted in the U.S. and other countries. The common expectation is that clinicians give diagnoses fundamentally based on the symptomatic and statistical manual called DSM-IV-TR. Furthermore, since the patient showed a melancholia-affinitive personality, as defined by Telenbach, H., a prescription of antidepressants, accompanied by supportive psychotherapy, would be the expected treatment, as is common in the case of a diagnosis of major depression.

At the beginning of the diagnosis and treatment, symptomatic and statistical diagnoses based on DSM-IV-TR were taken priority over the observation term, but, this case was diagnosed as depressive state of borderline personality disorder by reviewing the medical history sheet, after long time from the first medical examination.

Once the case was diagnosed as depressive state of borderline personality disorder, it might be commonly known that Olanzapine was to be prescribed for this case.

When a pathological situation, defined as the coexistence of an "angel personality" and a "devil personality," show only one side—the "angel" side—it could be difficult for a clinician to see that the exact diagnosis is a depressive state based on a borderline personality disorder. In such cases, psychiatric specialists (everywhere in the world) need to remember to see human beings as whole human beings. When specialists try to see their clients as whole human beings, they will easily see the clients' psychopathology. Every human being has walked his life accompanied with psychopathological problems.

Today, many reports are available confirming that Olanzapine is seriously effective for melancholia-affinitive depressions. The case described here should be included in this body of evidence. Since recently, the melancholia-affinitive personality has come to be thought of as a personality disorder, which indicates that the depressive state of borderline personality disorder could be included into same category.

In any event, it will be speculated that Olanzapine is extremely effective against depressive states based on personality disorders (33).

Olanzapine: 42cases

In the following cases, we see a mono-prescription of Olanzapine. Usually, the simplest case, like schizophrenia by DSM-IV-TR standards, should be introduced as a typical case. But my recent retrospective research showed me how many different situations and disorders exist that are effectively treated with Olanzapine. In other words, it was clarified that cases that are diagnosed simply as schizophrenia rarely exist. All the cases presented in this study—42 cases of 42 cases—represented different situations, not just simple schizophrenia.

Of course, simple schizophrenias in DSM-IV-TR were observed by according to symptomatic and statistical classification. But when psychopathological research and discussion was taken in to consideration, it was difficult to classify them into each diagnosis. These cases presented much evidence that the symptomatic and statistical criteria known as DSM-IV-TR has classified human beings simply and mechanically, and is really not an appropriate diagnostic tool for classifying actual, suffering human beings.

Since it is not within the scope of this text to describe all 42 cases in this study, I would like to introduce some cases that are impossible to diagnose, such as schizophrenia in psychopathological philosophy, in spite of the diagnosis guidelines suggested in DSM-IV-TR, which is a symptomatologic diagnostic manual.

From these observations, it is my wish that the importance and the effectiveness of Olanzapine will be understood.

Case 1. 26-year-old, female, a part-timer worker

History of illness and treatment: The young woman visited my psychiatric clinic for the first time when she was17 years old. Her medical records at the time showed that it was difficult for her to go to school due to "abdominal pain and headaches," but only in the morning. She stayed in bed until noon. When her mother forced her to go to school, she cried. Since she was absent from school three or four days a week, her mother, who was a teacher, suggested that she visit me.

When tested, the young girl showed 62 points on the SDS (Self-Rating Depression Scale by Zung), which is high. At the time, her doctor had prescribed Clomipramine 10mg twice a day. (SSRIs were not permitted at that time.)

After some time in a weekly psychotherapy situation, she was able to go to school.

One day, she was scouted as a photography model for a magazine for young people, and so she rapidly became the idle of young readers. But because the magazine was published only once a month, and because of low pay, she did not really have sufficient work. Still, she loved being praising so she decided to enter a photo model school. She went to school every day except when she was working as a model, which was highly estimated at the school. Any students was given an excused absence to work as a model.

After some time, she found work modeling at night, consequently, she often returned home as late as midnight. After the work, a photographer or his assistant, drove her home.

One day, the photographer, in a respectful and admiring voice, told her something flattering, and asked her to model nude for him. Without a second though, she accompanied him to a motel, and it was only after he raped her that she understood his real intention. But her told her that to the extent that she "accepted him" in the future, her situation as a model would be only for the better.

It was too late to return to a more innocent situation. She, who was brought up in the lap of luxury, continued the sexual relationship with deep conflict.

After several days, she could not sleep and could not rise from bed in the morning. And suddenly, she was saying to others things like: "I have a liaison with the famous talent, Mr. X. Do you envy me? He always accompanies me everywhere I go." "You know me? I am known by people all over the world." "You love me? I love you." "Where do you stay? Oh, Europe! Good! I wish to meet you—only your voice. Come here! As I am known widely, you will be able to find me." "Hello, do you associate with me? Let's make love."

When she visited me, she seemed precisely schizophrenic, based on her symptomatolgy. I immediately gave her an intravenous injection of Haloperidol and prescribed the same medicine in tablet form.

Furthermore, she often cried and said, "Mr. X is always watching me, but I cannot see him. Mr.X said to me, only he can watch me.

Next month, as he plans a big show in Tokyo, I am invited by him to participant as a model."

Such hallucination and delusion has continued for more than three years, accompanied by regressive behavior. She has actually passed most of her life in bed.

At that time, fortunately, the prescription of Olanzapine was officially permitted. Since she was diagnosed as schizophrenic, based on the symtomatic diagnostic manual, DSM-IV-TR, she was immediately given a prescription of Olanzapine 10mg. As a result, she showed astonishingly fast improvement, along with obesity due to over eating. Her body weight increased more than 20kg. But once she recovered from her psychological difficulties, she began to make efforts to reduce her weight until she arrived to an average body weight, which she has maintained after four continuous years of taking Olanzapine 10mg.

At the same time, some strange opinions became manifest amount some of treatment staff. For example; when a patient is determined to have reached remission, the patient must be released from psychotherapy sessions at the clinic.

I could never accept this opinion because the clinic staff is not treating a machine, but a whole human being, who is never simple. Nevertheless, the release opinion prevailed.

When I informed the patient that she would be finishing her therapy sessions, she told me that she still has anxiety, and she requested that I permit her to continue visiting the clinic and continue receiving psychotherapy treatments.

She still visits the clinic regularly and receiveds counseling and psychotherapy, saying, "I do not have enough confidence to leave here. Please, give me the authorization to continue as usual. I believe I need this support for the rest of my life."

She found work at a French restaurant, and continued work for several years, taking Olanzapine 10mg every day. She was absent only one day, and that was due to common a cold and high temperature.

Today, she is working at the restaurant as a star employee. Especially during holidays, many of guests visit the restaurant because of her good service. Nevertheless, she still complains that she has not enough confidence to continue the work, and she implores me to never reduce her dosage of Olanzapine. She has become a healthy girl, but she has never missed an appointment at the clinic for over five years.

Short discussion on this case: It would be difficult to clarify the appropriate and accurate diagnosis for this girl according to the symptomological criteria outlined in the DSM-IV-TR, since she has demonstrated a variety of symptoms, depending on her situation and state of mind.

If her school refusal was diagnosed as an episode that signaled the beginning of schizophrenia, it makes no sense that only Clomipramine 20mg could have led the case to even a simple improvement, never mind remission of schizophrenia. But, of course, her school refusal was not only a simple episode through the whole course of the illness. It is common knowledge that Clomipramine causes schizophrenia to become even worse, instead of improvement. It is more logical to recognize that her school refusal was never only the precursor of schizophrenia, but also her simple episode in adolescence. There has never been shown that schizophrenia is improved or prevented by Clomipramine, as far as I am aware.

The patient's second episode, showing hallucination and delusion, might be diagnosed as schizophrenia according to DSM-IV-TR. But, it is nevertheless suspicious that the patient not only rejected the treatment altogether, but also persisted in her requests of help from me and the treatment staff at my clinic. Of course, I am aware that schizophrenics do not always reject treatment, as contrasted with schizoaffective disorders. Furthermore, the schizophrenia may not be recognized as acute for as much as three years, but is usually regarded as a chronic stage, accompanied with systematized and adhered pathologic symptoms.

But, in this case, the patient improved dramatically with Olanzapine 10 mg, and returned to normal society while continuing the same dosage of Olanzapine, together with losing weight and returning from obesity to her normal body weight.

This case demonstrates the powerful effect of Olanzapine as evidence. I will, nevertheless, have to acknowledge that this patient might have recovered not only because of Olanzapine and therapy, but also with the continuous supportive association of her family, as well as the owner and staff of the restaurant, although schizophrenia is thought to be hard to deal with after a build-up of episodes. Furthermore, in this case use was never made of any social facilities because such facilities could never give the patient any suitable support and help. As a result, I could not help recognizing the contribution of Olanzapine to her recovery.

From these observation, we could speculate that her current situation depends on the A10 nerve work of Olanzapine. At any rate, we can certainly conclude that Olanzapine works for this patient in her particular life style and personality.

Although this case has been prescribed with simply Olanzapine, she is never diagnosed as schizophrenia. Based on the whole discussion, we will have to conclude that her diagnosis is a psychopathological adolescent crisis.

Freud, S. already argued that anyone who experiences overwhelming mental disorders from birth to adolescence fits his argument. This patient suffered from serious mental disorders due to her pathogenesis, but after the rigors of adolescence, she returned to health and entered into new society (34).

Case 2. 45-year-old male, administrative position in large company

Personality before illness: sparing no effort to maintain public order, workaholic, strict with his subordinates, highly esteemed for his work by his superiors.

Course of illness and treatment: He was an able employee since he entered the company. He had got a promotion to subsection chief at 30 years old, being promoted over the heads of his colleagues. Although his position was equal to section chief in other big companies, all employees were taking the reins of the company by laying down a multitude of managerial positions. So he was able to get a promotion to a head of the department after a promotion of the practical head of the department, and so on. But, when he was promoted to head of the department, similarly, he was eligible to get a promotion to executive.

He made it his policy to maintain public order in the company above all. He never forgave any mistake of his subordinates. Whenever his subordinate made a mistake in the work, he always levied punishment under the penal regulations, allowing no exceptions. And when he put all responsibility to errors on his supervisees; he never permitted them to get help from others. So it is not unexpected that his section always caused friction with others. He always said, "Since the opinions of superiors are correct, it is strictly enforced that the subordinates follow their judgment." As a result, there were few disputes in t he office.

He was always defensive and never joked, similar to a person who was educated by Confucianism. He never smoked or drank; he always read books and studied hard.

Due to his esteemed working style and excellent results, he was unexpectedly promoted to chief of the department. This was shocking to his colleagues and subordinates. And as soon as he was promoted to the chief of department, he became unsparing, not only to the subsection chief, but to everyone under him, more than before. He never smiled, and was always working without any rest.

It was natural that when his area of responsibility expanded, he worked harder. However he knew no fatigue, though he was probably growing tired gradually. But he never showed his tiredness

Although all his routine health examinations showed hypertension from the first, he ignored the directions of the company doctors and continued to work as much and as hard as when he first entered in the company.

After about a year as chief of his department, he was encouraged to take a holiday due to a business slump in the company. It had been a very long time since he had taken such a holiday, and in the middle of his vacation, he began to feel tired all the time and it was difficult for him to get up. He wondered if he was suffering from some disease so he consulted a doctor, who told him that he was probably fatigued from his work, and the doctor advised a rest. But he doubted the doctor's opinion. "This is a strange doctor," he said, "and I never am tired. I think this doctor is wrong. I think I have a serious disease."

At last, he visited the hospital in a medical school. Although he had a thorough checkup of all his organs and systems, all the doctors informed him similarly—that he was suffering only from essential hypertension, and they wanted to prescribe some medicines.

But, when he returned to his work, even though he did take the prescribed medicine, he was unable to perform as before. However strongly he tried to show strength, he did not do anything and, although he was able to go to his office as before, he did not work anymore. And in the next days, not only work was he unable to perform his work, but he felt he was losing his mind, so he came, by himself, to the medical office in the company.

He complained to his superiors that several doctors found no pathology by a thorough examination just a few days before, so what could be happening to his body? And the industrial doctor told him that he could be exhausted neurologically, and he provided the patient with a referral letter to me.

At the first examination, he had a defiant attitude from the first. As soon as he came into the examination room, he shouted that he is perfectly sane and that whatever medicine I prescribe, he will never take it. Possibly, he perceived that I was younger than he, so he spoke to me in an authoritative tone. But I spoke with him quietly, and I suggested that he was probably too exhausted to work, and that some treatments would be a good idea.

He immediately changed his attitude to something more receptive, but then suddenly showed anger. It was clear that he was confused and ambivalent. As we continued talking, his complaints gradually became illogical and contradictory. It was difficult to keep him tranquil, if only for short a interval. So when he seemed in a restful phase, I immediately gave him an Olanzapine 5mg lozenge to suck, accompanied with a prescription for the same medicine. Then, he began slowly to talk to me and tell me that he would like to take the medicine regularly and to recover his health.

The next morning, he called me to complain that he could sleep for only three hours. He felt the medicine was too weak, so I suggested him that he take two instead of one of the tablets of Olanzapine 5mg, and he agreed, but I did not hear from him for two weeks after taking Olanzapine 10mg.

After two weeks, he came to me and thanked me. He said he took the medicine and rested for two weeks, and now he feels great and he will not take the medicine anymore. I immediately asked him to wait a minute. I reminded him that he had been exhausted for more than ten years, and it is definitely premature to return to your work and to discontinue the medication, and that, furthermore, he should definitely continue receiving therapy treatments. But, he did not agree, and he did not come for his treatments.

According to the medical letter I provided for him, he had to take a rest for a month, but he ignored this and went to his office every day. His superiors considered his treatment plan, but they decided to allow him to work so that they would be assured order in his department. He completely returned to his office.

Short discussion of this case: This case showed recovery only by taking Olanzapine 10mg for two weeks and two week's rest. After returning to work, the patient showed no relapse; he may be in complete remission.

It was difficult to make an exact diagnosis for this patient because he recovered in only two weeks with Olanzapine 10mg and rest. He could be diagnosed as schizoaffective disorder since it was observed that he suffered mainly from a sudden disturbance of consciousness and a specific obsessive syndrome, as well as loss of memory. Furthermore, his sleeplessness and tension could be related to the onset of illness.

Due to the uncertainty of his diagnosis by use of DSM-IV-TR, he could be diagnosed as "atypische Psychosenbild (atypical psychosis:

Pauleikhoff, B.)" or "episodische Psychose (an episodic psychosis)," which was the single episode.

It has been well documented that such a pathogenetic situation can easily reverse itself. But it is undeniable that the patient recovered and went into with Olanzapine 10mg, even though he took this medicine for only two weeks. Consequently, Olanzapine showed dramatic effectiveness in this case.

Case 3. 6-year-old male

Course of illness and treatment: He grew up in free and uninhibited home. His parents gave him anything he wanted, and any behavior was permitted. For example, when he wished to have an expensive toy, his mother immediately went to a toy shop to get it for him; if the toy was unavailable at that shop, she went to another toy shop, even if it was a long distance from home.

When the child entered kindergarten, he gradually began to make trouble for the teachers. When he noticed something he disliked, he became suddenly angry and eve violent. At first, the teachers recognized his violent behavior as a first period of the rebellious phase, and they did not take his behavior seriously. But, the child hated to be directed by anyone, and whenever his teachers tried to lead him to return to the classroom, he ignored their orders and went off to play by himself.

Since the teachers were not permitted to leave him alone, they requested other kindergarten pupils to invite him to return, but when they tried to invite him, he became angry and hit his classmates with a stick. As soon as the teachers saw his violence, they tried to force him to quit his violent behavior, and he responded by throwing sand at their faces, especially their eyes. It was difficult for them to see, so they cried for help. But the child grasped the opportunity to jab them in the ribs. The teachers could not help running away from him, for fear of their safety.

At last, there was nothing to do but call in all the employees in the kindergarten and hold the child down.

The child's behavior continued to degenerate. Once, he held hair of a little girl in his class and pulled her around; another time, he pierced another child's head with the pencil. The teachers all realized that this violent behavior went far beyond a simple rebellious phase. So the child's mother was called in to discuss the matter with the teachers as well as the principal and the supervising teacher of the school. The child was also present at the meeting.

In the middle of the discussion, the child complained that he wanted a certain toy, and immediately the mother answered that she would be happy to buy the toy after the meeting, and she asked him to be quiet. In response, he suddenly threw a chair at one of the teachers.

The mother responded to this by quietly asking the boy to behave, but he did not behave. He threw chairs and desks, and even the principal could not be approachable to him. At last, the meeting and discussion were so disrupted, it was terminated.

Hereafter the violence of the child's behavior became ever more severe and more frequent. He began to smash windowpanes and to use the broken class to inflict injury to the faces of his female classmates. This kind of behavior surfaced every time the child found himself in an environment that was outside his comfort zone.

It was not long before the parents of the other children in the kindergarten began to complain and to demand that the child be expelled from the kindergarten if his behavior could not be brought under immediate control.

So the principal informed the parents that they would have to seek professional psychological treatment for the child, or else he would be expelled from the kindergarten.

However, the child's father maintained that it is natural for a child to be given freedom. He said that all children must act wild to work off excess energy, and so the boy should be set free. The mother felt caught between the point of view of her husband and the concerns of the other parents. And, of course, the father never listened to the parents of the other children in the class.

The mother, who was totally perplexed, visited the author to get suggestions, and she made the child accept a meeting with me.

At the first examination, the child was able to talk with me and the other psychologist quietly, even though some troubled information was gathered from the interview. I told he mother that I would like to perform play therapy with the child, and that I would like to prescribe some appropriate medication, and the mother immediately agreed. She told me that she would not be able to return home if she didn't bring a prescription with her.

My initial and subsequent examinations of the child let me to diagnose him with borderline personality disorder.

When the child was in my therapy room, he talked and played like an angel, so it was hard for me to believe what I had been told about his behavior in the kindergarten.

However, at the next appointment, the psychotherapist who was in charge of the child's case burst into my room and announced that it is impossible to treat the child with play therapy. From the beginning of the therapy, he began destroying things, then he smashed all the windowpanes, one after another, and he attacked the doctor with pieces of broken glass. The doctor was reluctant to even be in the same room with this child.

But, when I went into the play room, the child immediately changed his demeanor and, in the voices of an angel, he asked, gently and softly, "Why did you come into the room, doctor? I promised my mother I would go shopping with her for two toys." But as soon as I left the room, he immediately became violent, again.

I rushed into the room and demanded of the child, "Do you promise to take some medicine from tonight?" He answered gently, "OK! I will take the medicine."

My diagnosis was borderline personality disorder, and I decided to prescribe Olanzapine 2.5mg, with the informed consent of his mother. But, the next morning the mother called me and said the medicine was too weak to controllable the boy, and she asked permission to increase the dose. I asked her to wait for a week, since the patient is a young child."

In this connection, the child received a thorough examination in the department of brain surgery and neurology, including a child-welfare consultation, but nothing abnormal was found.

The mother could not wait until the next week, however, and she gave the boy 5mg of Olanzapine. Unfortunately, although she gave him Olanzapine 5mg, he cut the face of a classmate, and the scar from this injury will remain with her through her life. After this incident, his mother immediately came to me complaining that Olanzapine 5mg is not effective, and she urged me to elevate the dosage. She assured me that no side effects had appeared and that she had come to me with the blessing of her husband.

At that point, I agreed with her and I prescribed Olanzapine 10mg. Within three months on this dosage of Olanzapine, the child's violent outbursts had been reduced to about one in a month.

With consistent sessions of play therapy, the child gradually came to play in an age-appropriate style. As long as he plays in the therapeutic context, he behaves as a normal child without any violent behavior and emotional excitement.

Now, this child is ready to enter the school. Unfortunately, although he was permitted to enter the school, his classmates avoid him because they heard of his violent behaviors in kindergarten. As a result, he is always isolated in the school. Although he wishes to play with his classmates, no one wants to approach him. When he tries to approach them, they run away, so he raises his voice, "Hey! Play with me!" But, no one, not even the teacher on duty, responds to him.

His mother and father are aware of this situation, which they understand, and they are looking for a new school where his history won't follow him so he can make a fresh start.

Short discussion: There is evidence to suggest a diagnosis of borderline personality disorder in this case; it fits the definition outlined in DSM-IV-TR. The only problem is the age of the child. Usually, the growth of brain function and anatomical identifications are not integrated in the average three-year-old. We can speculate that the child has grown to his age without any conductor in his brain. In fact, the response to Olanzapine showed the evidence of his brain functions. In other word, the result showed his abnormalities.

Although Olanzapine is not a normal solution for young children, the results with this child were very promising; he seemed to be cured of his seriously problematic behavior, and without any disturbance or side effects to his organs, including not only the liver, but also kidneys, pancreas and blood.

Reports are available that show good results for Olanzapine and changing the disorderly behavior of young children, but, as far as I know, there are no long-term studies of effectiveness and safety of Olanzapine for young children. Such studies will have to be performed because many of children could be saved by this drug.

In the meantime, I have tried on a number of occasions to reduce the dosage of Olanzapine for this child, but the reduced prescription immediately returns the child to his previous violent behavior, so I have prescribed the same dosage of Olanzapine for him on an ongoing basis. His parents have not complained. In fact, they (as well as teachers) have requested an even higher dose because of the child's occasional outbursts of violence, but I have not raised the dose because no one knows what effect such a dose could have on the child.

The social pathogeneses of this kind of case also warrants discussion. This child's teachers and other peripheral people treated him as a problem child after only one case of violent behavior, and they have continued to regard him as a problem child even when his behavior changed dramatically. The reaction of peripheral societies can actually cause a child to perform as they expect him to perform. And this is an issue that can confound the good effect of medicine or any other therapy.

In addition, this child's family background influences his behavior. The child was born and grew up in an antisocial family environment, created not only by his parents, but also by his grandparents.

In any event, this child has a right to live in this society, and it has been confirmed that Olanzapine helped and supported him to do so.

Case 4. 48-year-old male, an executive of a large Japanese company

Personality before illness: social, precise, considerate, well-ordered.

Course of illness and treatment: He was the hope of the president of the company. He was very good at human relationships, and has a deep consideration of the company's employees, as well as the employees of subcontractors. He was a huge asset to the company.

His daughter, who went to a university a long distance from home and so returned only every week ends, did not return home one weekend, and no one could find out why or where she was. without for the first without any information. She also did not return home on the following day, so the family called repeatedly to her cell phone, but the phone was cut off from power.

Although her father and her family made contacts with her friends, they were still unable to find out where she was or why she did had not come home. When there was still no word on Monday, the father called the university, but he could not get any information.

At last, her father asked the police to search for her, although he did not wish to think she had been involved in an accident. After three months, his father received a call from the police while he was in an important conference at work. The police wanted him to confirm the identity of a hand that had been found, separated from its body. "This is impossible to believe!" he shouted. He became confused in his brain, thinking about one after another possible situations.

Nevertheless, he arrived to the scene, accompanied by the policemen, and found the left hand with a ring, which was the ring he had given his daughter as a present after she passed her university exams. The father was stunned and was unable to speak. Yet, the coroner and a policeman rained questions on him about the hand, but before they could finish, he suddenly grasped and one of the policeman by the neck and shouted at them.

More than 10 policemen came around him and roughed him up with kicks and blows, and forced him to the ground and handcuffed him, then took him to the police station and put into a cell. For three days, the father sat in the cell and muttered to himself. He refused all food and water.

In time, the father hired a lawyer, who came to the jail and to secure is release, but the condition of the release was that the father receive a psychiatric evaluation. This is how I became involved in this case. The father arrived to my office in an official police car. By then, I had received the file on this man and I was already aware of the details of the case. As soon as the man, accompanied by his lawyer, entered my office, I offered him Olanzapine. I asked him to take a 10mg tablet, informing him that I already knew about his case and that the tablet would make him relaxed. I told him there was nothing to fear.

After taking the tablet, the man drank a cup of water straight down, and continued drinking water until he had consumed more than 500ml, then he slept deeply. snoring loudly.

The mother of the girl came to my office at the same time, and her condition was also not good. Whatever the lawyer asked her, she showed only a confused response. And so I prescribed for her Olanzapine 5mg. I thought her disturbance of consciousness was not as deep as her husband's since she didn't witness the scene directly. She willingly took the medicine by herself, and she left the clinic saying thanking everyone.

Without a doubt, these patients received daseinsanalysis (see References) consistently for over five years.

The father returned to his work and assumed an unimportant post, but after six months, he was promoted, and he became an executive in the company after one year. The mother, however, gained 26kg of weight and she began to show signs of diabetes mellitus. Because she needed medication for the diabetes, I had to take her off the Olanzapine because Olanzapine is not permitted to diabetes mellitus patients in Japan. The mother implored me to find a way for her to continue with the Olanzapine. She said she believed that her "mind and spirit would die without the Olanzapine," and based on this, and other things the woman had said to me, I became concerned that suicide could be in her thoughts.

In my professional judgment, this woman should have continued on the Olanzapine as well as her prescription for diabetes mellitus. This combination of medicines is not prohibited in the U.S. and other countries. Yet, I was not prepared to go against the law in my country. "Give me two months," I said to the woman. "I will help you overcome the diabetes mellitus. This is the only way you will be able to return to your prescription of Olanzapine in Japan." The woman agreed reluctantly. She said she wanted her lawyer to join our discussion. I explained to the lawyer that I would like to honor the woman's request and I would like to break the law for her life, since Olanzapine could protect her from suicide. But I cannot, so I ask that you and she accept my terms—that she reduce her body weight by two kg in a week, and 20 kg after two months. Furthermore, you make her bring down her blood sugar by use of my diet plan.

The lawyer answered that he would like to make the woman obey my plan, and that he would try to protect me and her from any disturbance. After two months, the mother's body weight returned to 50 kg and her blood sugar was within an acceptable range.

For more than five years, now, both husband and wife have continued taking Olanzapine, along with therapy sessions with me. After working with this couple, I believe that their behavior was natural, considering their psychic trauma and deep mourning over the terrible fate of their daughter.

Short discussion: Needless to say, the case is diagnosed as psychic traumatic stress disorder (PTSD). Unfortunately, no treatment method is available in the symtomatic diagnostic manual, DSM-IV-TR. Furthermore, this couple who experienced such a rare psychic trauma will have to be treated most carefully. It is possible that cognitive scientific treatments would drive them to suicide. As a result, it is my belief that only Olanzapine (along with daseinsanalysis) made them turn to the future, in spite of SSRIs and cognitive behavior therapy (41) (42).

At the beginning of this study, I did not suspect that there would be such a large number of patients who were treated at first by Olanzapine, continued taking Olanzapine, and recovered by Olanzapine. Added to this number the schizophrenic patients who were diagnosed based on psychopathology, then treated by Olanzapine, and the total number of patients who achieved recovery through this drug is huge.

The details of these studies will be discussed at chapter V.

Chapter V. Discussion

Introduction

I performed the retrospective investigation on the 453 cases prescribed Olanzapine at the Department of Psychiatry, Jozuka Mental Clinic. Results clarified that the medicine has wide effects, for example, Multiacting Receptor Targeted Antipsychotic (MARTA). It was interesting that the typical strong points of this medicine were effective for depression of typus melancholicus, which is thought to be an SSRI effective disorder, and for chronic fatigue syndrome-like schizophrenia. Furthermore, it was recognized as a matter off interest, that Olanzapine was very effective even for children from age six.

It is seriously speculated that Olanzapine could elevate Beta-endorphins and encephalin in the A10 nerves of the brain, due to evidence of improvement of negative symptoms in schizophrenia.

Both disorder and disease might be taken ill through exhausted situations.

Consequently, we must conclude that Olanzapine is effective for all of these disorders.

Indications of Olanzapine by Country

Figure 8, below, shows official indications of Olanzapine by country. The indications of Olanzapine are not only schizophrenia (except for Japan), but also depressions in many countries. It is expected that depressions were classified into indications of Olanzapine because of MARTA.(35) It might seem strange that borderline personality disorders are not classified into these indications of Olanzapine, but it is not yet clear whether Olanzapine has a precise effect on borderline personality disorder.(36)(37)

U.S.A	Schizophrenia, acute mixed and manic episodes in Bipolar I Disorder, Bipolar depressive episode, Refractory Depression (+SSRI)
Canada	Schizophrenia and related disorders, manic and depressive mixed state in Bipolar I Disorder, Bipolar I manic state, mixed state maintenance treatment
Europe	Schizophrenia, medium to heavy manic disorder
Australia	Schizophrenia and related disorders, acute mixed and manic episodes in Bipolar I Disorder, Bipolar I manic disorder, mixed state, prevention against relapse into manic state
Japan	Schizophrenia

Figure 8: Indications of Olanzapine by country

Since this is a retrospective study, there were no arbitrary prescriptions of Olanzapine in those cases. A number of non-effective cases by prescription of approved indications of each medicine were also shown. Observation led us to conclude that in this study any treatment by a diagnosis based on symptomatology is meaningless.

It was understood that the indication of Olanzapine was officially schizophrenia in each country. But, when the special feature, such as MARTA and A10 selective work were considered in psychiatry, psychoneurotic pharmacology was favored over clinical psychiatry. Or, it is suspected that economics was considered over practice.

In any case, indications must be expanded, depending on the dosage of Olanzapine, whether the form is zydis tablet or usual tablet and powder.

Usually, since it has not been clarified whether the indicated form was zydis tablets or ordinary tablets in almost all reports to date, as far as I know, it has been a long time since doctors, including me, have not been able to know the facts. Because, the official permits have been issued after the consumption of the previous type Olanzapine.

It might be seemed strange that I have discussed such a situation. Researchers tested the effect of Olanzapine using different forms of tablets, but intra venous dosages of Olanzapine could well differ from the effects of tablets. As a result, it might be thought that indications of Olanzapine are different country by country.

In any case, it is likely that, everywhere, the economic principle will prevail over the importance of treating human beings. However high the development of psycho-pharmacological studies might be in a given country, that country will have to be considered a backward nation if the official indication of Olanzapine is only schizophrenia.

Limits of Treatment Made by DSM-III Diagnoses, Effects of Olanzapine

Today, the symtomatic and statistical diagnostic manual has been commonly invited into clinical practices. However, as we have seen from the results of this study, contemporary diagnostic methods by use of the manual never include life histories or life styles of the patients.

When DSM-III was first published in the world, members of the American Psychiatric Association emphasized that the manual was intended as a guide for all specialists to classify all psychiatric diseases into the greatest common measure and statistical classification. It was stressed that the manual was not suitable for clinical practice or to express the general condition of individual cases.

It was not anticipated that symtomatic and statistical diagnostic classifications would be invited into a clinical sense and became a fundamental diagnostic average. Nevertheless, the diagnostic method by use of this classification became common. In reality, however, it is impossible (in this study) that the initial diagnosis in a specific case would prevail throughout the life of the treatment.

Switched from Olanzapine to Aripirazol

In this retrospective investigation, there were 54 cases of Olanzapine switched to Aripirazol. Of these clients, 83% (39 of the 54) were diagnosed with schizoaffective disorder, and the remaining 15 cases were diagnosed with beginning of schizophrenia.

The prescription method is thought to be the typical method to treat schizophrenia today. In this situation, I recognized that this method was not only the prescription for schizophrenia, but also for schizoaffective disorder, as mentioned above.

Schizoaffective disorder has been classified into two categories: (1) A mixed state of schizophrenia and manic depressive illness (mixed psychosis), and (2) independent psychotic syndrome.

Kleist, K. had named the latter syndrome "degenerative psychosis" and "peripheral psychosis." These psychoses were classified into "atypical psychosis (atypische Psychose)" by Leonhard, K., studied under Kleist, K.

He noted the distinctive features as follows: (1) acute onset, course of illness is phased and periodic, and good prognosis without serious defect; (2) disturbance of consciousness, emotional and psychomotor function, accompanied with serious sensory hallucinations and fluctuating delusions differing from schizophrenia; (3) pre-onset personality characterized as irritable, precise and stubborn, differing from the autistic personality of schizophrenia; (4) mental or somatic moment commonly observed at onset.

Leonhard classified these disease groups into "cycloid psychosis" (zykloide Psychose) and "atypical psychosis" (atypische Schizophrenie) from the perspective of the pathological situation and clinical genetics. Psychomotor disease, derangement psychosis and anxiety-ecstatic psychosis belong to the former, and emotional abundant paraphrenia, cycloid catatonia and schismatic speech disorder belong to the latter.

Although the independence of atypical psychosis was still not clarified, Leonhard argued the independence of atypical psychosis from the studies of clinical genetics by research into a line of decent. But Mitsuda and Kurosawa argued the differentiation between the typical group and the atypical group by comparative clinical genetics saying that each atypical psychosis showed not only phenomenological changes but also genetically independent diseases by treating an independent atypical psychosis differ from typical psychosis (i.e. schizophrenia). As a result, they declined to treat atypical psychosis as a transition form between typical and atypical groups.

Hatotani, T. had speculated on these groups as a congenital functional reduction between midbrain and pituitary line from the viewpoint of somato-pathological ideation, including endocrinological ideation. Mitsuda argued these situations in relation to epilepsy.

Descriptions and reports about atypical psychosis had been available in German and French psychiatry. Ey, H. classified chronic psychoses as pathological personalities (la pathologie de la personnalite) and acute psychoses as pathological conscious situations (la pathologie de la conscience) . The former would be recognized as typical schizophrenia and the latter would be recognized as atypical psychosis (33).

Compared to the German definition, the clinical borderline between a narrow-sense schizophrenia in an endogenous (functional) psychoses and a manic depressive illness in the U.S. is not always clear. Atypical psychosis has been called an unidentified psychosis group, which seems the same as a mixed psychosis.

The psychosis has an acute or sub-acute appearance, and the severity of emotional undulation, along with hallucination and delusion, improves within a short term with good prognosis. Spontaneous appearance is possible, but usually the psychosis appears due to psychosomatic stress. Some cases show reversible functional disturbance of the limbic system, midbrain-pituitary grand and abnormalities of epileptic electro-encephalic-graph. Some of the diagnoses in DSM-IV and ICD-10 coincide with the atypical psychosis.

The concept of atypical psychosis developed psychopathologically mainly in Germany and Japan. As a result, atypical psychosis was defined as an identified psychosis group with peripheral features of the big three psychoses: schizophrenia, manic-depressive illness, and epilepsy as illustrated in Figure 9 below. But, in fact, some psychiatrists raise objections to this opinion.

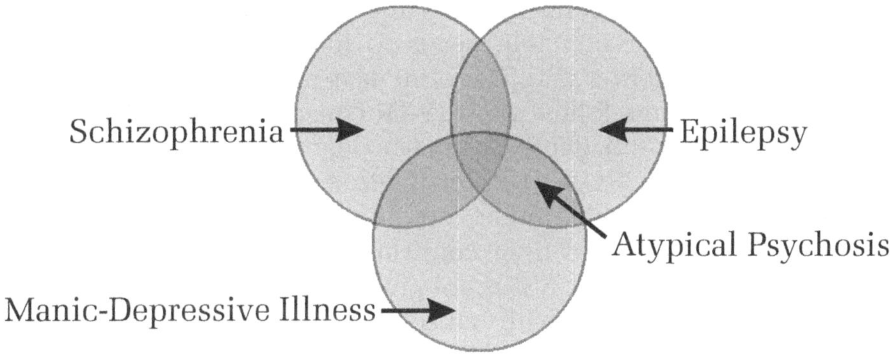

Figure 9: Aytypical Psychosis

Here, some clinicians are in favor of switching from Olanzapine to Aripirazol in order to improve the depressive state in schizophrenic patients. But such a method is not needed for patients who have the possibility to improve by the antidepressant effect of Olanzapine.

Both Olanzapine and Aripirazol have distinctive side effects. For example, it is commonly thought that Olanzapine invites a sugar-metabolic disorder. Let us consider this possibility: schizophrenic patients are commonly thin because of their disease, even if they eat a lot. We much consider that as the treatment develops, they may become obese as a rebound of a self-preservation instinct of a living body. And Aripirazol is sometimes associated with an instability similar to an akathisia-like behavior. In such a situation, therefore, clinicians should proceed with caution when considering a switch from

Olanzapine to Aripirazol. Such switching of treatments might be wrong or worse for patients.

Switched from Olanzapine to Olanzapine + Aripirazol to Olanzapine alone

The next change of prescription forms was investigated on 50 cases. This course of prescriptions is thought to be more common than the previous style discussed.

But, after examining some of the cases, it was shown that the common prescription was not always commonly indicative of the case. Atypical psychosis was also present in indicative cases, although—even today—it is not clear whether the psychosis is a peripheral type of schizophrenia or a developed condition of depression, though it is clear that sufferers of the psychosis demonstrate a disturbance of consciousness and confusion. But it is commonly observed that at beginning stages of the psychosis look similar to a typical major depression that develops into atypical psychosis or schizoaffective disorder within several days or weeks.

When clinicians follow DSM-IV-TR conscientiously, all of these disorders would be diagnosed as major depression. Thus, beginners usually prescribe SSRI or SNRI for the first choice for patients, who are emotionally unstable. In fact, not only beginners but also experienced clinicians often fail to confirm the level of consciousness before diagnosing. When SSRIs are given to a patient suffering from depression, the SSRIs usually make him worse; due to the SSRIs' activate effects. In the past, antidepressants, accompanied with slight suppressive antipsychotics like Perphenazine, were prescribed for depression of reduced consciousness. At that time, only beginners would prescribe single medicines. After gaining experience, some clinicians prescribed more than three medicines in consideration of synergistic effects to secure better effectiveness and reduce harmful side effects.

However, it is now commonly thought that a single-prescription is better than a combination of medicines. And, in any case, since it is difficult to confirm which method is the best, a single-medicine approach is probably best.(37)

Olanzapine readily corresponds to the clinical situation of A10 nerve disturbance.

A10 nerves in tegmentum of midbrain are connected with midbrain, amygdalold nucleus (related to emotion, fear, adaptability), hippocampus, basal ganglia (related to somatic motor), nucleus accumbens (related to limbic system, called emotional and visceral brain) and frontal association area (related to personality, movement, motivation and plan), and make a good feeling in human beings by the secretion of Dopamine.

The amygdalold nucleus judges an individual's likes and dislikes, and the basal ganglia express the result of judgments through the face muscles. The nucleus accumbens rise up volition, and the fovea cortex gives a supremely good feeling and intellectual good feeling in the frontal association area. In these situations, the frontal association area secrets twice as much Dopamine as usual.(29)-(32)

Recently, it is speculated that the A10 nerves actually work as the conductor in individual brains.

From these phenomena, Olanzapine would be psycho-pharmacologically the most suitable medicine for clinicians whether they might be beginners or experienced specialists. Today, in fact, indications of Olanzapine are officially permitted for "schizophrenia and its peripheral diseases" in the whole world except for Japan.

When a clinician is confronted with a difficult-to-diagnose client, he would be advised to prescribe Olanzapine at onset. Then, if necessary, after taking a rest, the client will be able to improve by additional SSRIs.

It might be easy to diagnose major depressions, but it would be difficult to give exact diagnoses in other depressions. But a course of medication that includes Olanzapine and SSRI is waiting for official sanction from governments world wide. The case mentioned above seemed diagnostically to be a major depression, but, since slight disturbance of consciousness was observed, Olanzapine was prescribed and an additional agent to prevent falling into schizoaffective disorder.

Furthermore, the first period of thirty-year-old delusional state, which had already been forgotten in the diagnostic criteria and might be diagnosed as delusional disorder by symtomatic and statistical diaganostic criteria, should be investigated. Of course, the first period of thirty-year-old delusional state fundamentally differs from delusional disorder. The feature of this state is that the subject of the delusion is only one person (usually the husband) and never generalizes to other persons. The delusional idea is rarely acted upon. And usually the delusion subsides before age 40.

The case described in this study was a very rare case in terms of taking action based on delusional ideation. And I am doubtful about including this kind of pathological situation in schizophrenic disorders.

Some opinions and speculations are available on the phenomenon of a patient suffering from "the first period of thirty-year-old delusional state," as follows: the symptoms seem to appear at just the point when a wife and a husband are estranged for long term. Over time, delusion sometimes subsides because of the husband's response (or, sometimes, delusion is realized by a husband's response). A couple rarely seeks therapy unless some big trouble happens. Since this disorder deeply depends on the psychoenergy between husband and wife, the wife seeks therapy (or, more often, is brought to therapy) only when she acts on her delusion as if it is reality. Thus, it is difficult to know how many such patients exist, even in a small local area.

In the case in this study, the wife's delusions were triggered by a change in lifestyle when the children went to school and she had free time on her hands. She began to feel abandoned by her husband, who was ever more busy at his work. She was treated fundamentally by psychotherapy (including her husband), and was prescribed Olanzapine 5mg at first, increasing gradually to 10mg. The method was so-called family therapy. When her delusional ideation diminished, Aripirazol was added to recover her sexual desire, but afterward, I found that such a consideration was not needed.(38)(39)

First, SSRIs; switched to polymedicines; switched to Olanzapine: 90 cases.
AND
First, SSRIs; switched to polymedicines; switched to Aripirazol+ Olanzapine: 132 cases (include the 90 cases)

The prescription of SSRIs is commonly made for major depressions, anxiety disorders, obsessive compulsive disorders or social anxiety disorders based on the symptomatic and statistical diagnostic manual.

However, in the first course of prescriptions, at last improvement was observed with only Olanzapine. Although such changes had been difficult to anticipate, this phenomenon actually showed up in clinical situations when retrospective investigations were performed. Both courses may seem unacceptable in the usual prescriptive methods, when the investigations were prospective researches.

Some example are shown from actual situations, as follow: Some patients were diagnosed precisely as one of the disorders in DSM-III, mentioned above. But, as a number of problems were observed in DSM-III and under, many other medicines were invited to improve these problems. At last, due to the cases that clearly demonstrated the fundamental troubles and problems of borderline personality disorders, the cases improved by prescriptions of Olanzapine. In other cases, improvement was shown with Olanzapine, although the usual switching of the prescription to Aripirazol was performed first. Aripirazol was not effective but rather worsened, so Aripirazol was changed to Olanzapine, again. Needless to say, Olanzapine was effective for these patients.

Other strange, but common, cases are shown as follow:

Although the cases were diagnosed as the typical depression, and the patients recovered by prescription of only SSRIs, they were never advised—or prescribed—to take a rest, but immediately returned to work, sometimes harder than before, because they did not feel their diseases or the necessity of taking a rest. It should have been expected that they would relapse if they were on prescriptions of a single, low dose of SSRIs. Consequently, they requested more medicines, one after another, until they improved. At last, they became too exhausted to work. Although they did not sleep through the night, they hated sleepy sensation due to medications. They could not feel the differentiation between exhaustion and depressive mood. The personalities of such patients were usually Type A. These patients commonly requested a change of prescription or additional medicines. As a result, they would have to take a lot of medicines, but they would never improve. At last, they would have to be prescribed Olanzapine and rest, and to improve by force.

By the time they reached this stage in their recovery process, they had already become nonresponsive to high dosages and to many of the SSRIs and SNRIs. So therapists had little choice but to prescribe Olanzapine, which worked on selective A10 nerves.

As SSRIs do not commonly show clinical improvement to tiredness and exhaustion on most patients, the selective A10 work of Olanzapine is a more dependable way to improve these situations. It has been observed the fact that depression due to Type A behavior patterns has showed significant clinical improvement by use of Olanzapine. However, it usually takes time until before Olanzapine is prescribed for these patients because it is a typical Type A behavior pattern to desire improvement only by elevating the dosage of SSRIs and to request such dosage. Since there is an official upper limit to the permissible dosage of any single SSRI, these patients will have to take many kinds of SSRI to get their desired result. At last, they gradually recognize that they will never improve with SSRIs. They recognize there will be no way to improve other than rest and Olanzapine.

As a result of this time lapse, it is speculated that a number of such people have already fallen into a so-called Integration Disorder. There is some speculation that the interceptive effects of glutamic acid might be effective on such persons. Thus, the method of switching to Aripirazol might be meaningless, when, instead, switching to the interceptive effects of glutamic could work better.

In this kind of case, we suspect that an exhausted condition plus multiple medicines equal negative symptoms. (38)

Furthermore, although the patients were diagnosed with serious exhaustive depression, they want to feel good all the time. At the beginning of treatment, they were able to feel good (compared to how they felt before) by taking SSRIs, but the good feeling did not last. Some of these patients will improve with the selective A10 effects and the interceptive effect of glutamic acid as Olanzapine.

Although many of the patients in this category were not recognized as major depressives, they complained of depression and, indeed, they showed symptoms of depression at the first examination. Additionally, they usually requested a prescription of Aripirazol. Since selective A10 effects and interceptive effect of glutamic acid do not exist in Aripirazol, the patients cannot help depending on Olanzapine in the last analysis.

From these observations we have learned that depressions diagnosed by symptomology were not always major depressions, but depressive episodes showing major depression-like symptoms.

Dramatic Improvement with Olanzapine alone: 42 cases

The number of schizophrenic disorders in my clinic are few; nearly all patients were able to distinguish right from wrong.

The A10 nerves in the tegmentum of the midbrain are connected with the midbrain amygdaloidal nucleus (related to emotion, fear, adaptability), the hippocampus, basal ganglia (related to somatic motor), the nucleus accumbens (related to limbic system, referred to as the emotional and visceral brain), and the frontal association area (related to personality, movement, motivation, and planning). And the make a human being aware of a good feeling by the secretion of Dopamine.

The amygdalold nucleus judges an individual's likes and dislikes, and the basal ganglia expresses the result of these judgments through the face muscles. The nucleus accumbens raises up volition, and the fovea cortex provides emotional and intellectual feelings of well being in the frontal association area. The frontal association area secrets twice as much Dopamine as usual in these situations.(29)-(32). (See Figure 1, p. xref, Anatomy of A10 Nerve and Neurotransmission Systems)

Recent thinking allows the possibility that A10 nerves actually work as the conductor over the whole individual brain. Thus, there are too few patients who come to show a praecox feeling. As a result, it is speculated that all the areas in the brain, in most psychoses including schizophrenia, might be disturbed to integrate into the A10 nerves.(29)-(32).

The next type of case that responded to Olanzapine alone was the case of six-year-old child. Despite his uncommon behavior, he was not classified as a special type child, but a common type child. Since it is commonly shown in the mass media that even pre-kindergarten pupils are capable of performing vicious crimes, the case presented here is not so uncommon. This child's behavior was not treated as a criminal because of his parents' power and his family's support, but such as behaviors could surely be considered vicious crimes in common understanding.

I would like to investigate and analyze this phenomena clinically in terms of pediatric psychiatry.

The current childrearing theory that all children must be reared only by positive reinforcement and not by any outdated traditional ideas began to take hold all over the world from about 1975. At this time, the world gained a certain stability, not only economically, but also in international relationships. Since, before that, people had behaved according to the traditional customs of each country, they were surprised and bewildered to hear of such sudden changes in methods of childrearing, and they did not know how to make such a change. Because they reared their children according to traditional policy and teachings from the older generations, it was natural that they could not understand how to rear their children by the new methods. But they had to try to rear their children by praising and reinforcing positive behavior, anyway, even seriously inappropriate behaviors, because rearing of children by praising was the national policy. Parents reared their children in bewilderment and, of course, children were never scolded by parents or anyone else.

Until this time, children were thought to be relatively stable after the first stage of rebellion until the pre-puberty stage. But, children who grew up in this suddenly changed circumstance immediately turned into a mob of sorts, as evidenced by classroom disruptions, smoking, drinking and hazing. These situations were not considered pathogeneic.

Furthermore, borderline personality disorders were suddenly showing up in pre-pubescent children, and young borderline personality disorders easily turned into a mob. None of these were diagnosed as Asperger's disorder, for example, but just borderline personality disorder (39). Furthermore, governments and/or educational trends established by so-called experts in some countries forced a belief that there is no such thing as rebellious stages in child growth and development. Even the term disappeared from textbooks and from the practice of psychiatry and psychology.

As a result, young parents, who never knew the existence of rebellious stages, reared their own children only in bewilderment at the rebellious stages that, in fact, existed, whether the words appeared in text books or not. Even if they requested help from specialists, the only suggestion they would get is to watch silently and gently while their children grow.(40) This is especially a problem concerning the pre-pubescent rebellious stage, which is the formation period of personality, and is the brain's physiologically integrative stage.

Two problems developed: children did not get the guidance and structure they needed in order to pass successfully through the rebellious stages and become competent, integrated developing adults, so the incidence of assorted psychological difficulties increased in the population. At the same time, however, real diagnoses, such as schizophrenia, were not permitted. Only something vague like borderline personality disorder was permitted, which prevented any kind of meaningful treatment for a maladies that, basically, occurred in the first place only because of inappropriate child-rearing practices.

Although both schizophrenia cases and cases of borderline personality disorder could grow up in psycho-physiologically similar appearances, their situations could easily diverge as they reach adulthood, depending on the depth of of the pathogenesis. When these speculations were considered as the fundamental ideation, the most important medicine available could well be the selective A10 nerve work of Olanzapine.

In this light, the original disorder of the 42 cases that were dramatically and positively affected by Olanzapine make sense.

In the children studied, depressions similar to the depressions of typus melancholicus were found. These depressions showed more than 70 points on the SDS (Self-rating Depression Scale: Zung) and ketone body in urine, which is found only in serious diabetes mellitus or severe mental disorders accompanied with anxiety and exhaustion, or in autointoxication of psychosomatic disease in children. Their symptoms are characterized as follows: They can understand and answer 'Yes' or 'No' to therapists' questgions, instead of continuous crying. But, these disorders might not be diagnosed as schizoaffective disorder, and are not available in DSM-IV-TR.

But, Olanzapine was significantly effective for these disorders, which were difficult to classify, though they were similar to bipolar type-I manic-depressive mixed situation, but they did not show the manic state. Furthermore, they retained normal level of consciousness. They were able to respond for about three minutes, then fell into unintelligible conversation, as defined by Jaspers, K. When such symptoms were observed, medications would have to be performed immediately. And immediate improvement was observed with Olanzapine zydis tablets. These patients usually do not re-visit the clinic because they recovered by one tablet of Olanzapine. In fact, no retrospective research found their relapse in these patients. It was considered that these phenomena might be invited by the special character of Olanzapine.

In cases of posttraumatic stress disorder, such as Case 4, described above, of the couple whose daughter was mutilated, who would be able to heal his unforgettable psychic trauma? They experienced a sudden and unbelievably cruel trauma, as if their own bodies were cut and wounded. But t hey have been living together by taking Olanzapine. Olanzapine may have given them power to live, although they suffered a huge trauma of the heart, because of its effects on the A10 nerves. A trauma of the body body will recover after some days, but an emotional or mental trauma is often considered impossible to recover. But this husband and wife, who have continued to visit me, said, "We knew the medicines you prescribed are intended to treat schizophrenia. It's my joke that we are suffering from schizophrenia! But in any case, we will continue to take Olanzapine as long as we live, because Olanzapine is living in our hearts."

Some scientists might complain that such a description is not science. But, each therapist must decide whether he prefers to make a lifeless medicine into an organic agent, or to give an inorganic agent for patient as lifeless.(43)

Kimura, B. admonished psychiatrists: "Objective natural scientific decisions based on medicines' effects to intend non-subjective quantification is meaningless, when clinical decision on antipsychotics were performed. The only comprehensive anthropological discussion based on exact psychopathological consideration will be able to grasp the exact relationships between psychoses as human disease and medication by medical doctor as human being."

I recognized that contemporary psychiatrists who depend only on medications will have to learn and accept Kimura's admonition. Every psychiatrist will have to prescribe by making an inorganic agent to be a living agent for living patients. If contemporary psychiatrists accept Kimura's admonition, they will feel no responsibility of his prescription. However, the medicine could have unexpected possibilities, as with Olanzapine. Even until today, wide and deep possibilities of Olanzapine have already shown in clinical settings.

Indications of Olanzapine will have to be wider and deeper, based on these observations, considerations, and discussions.

Differences Between Schizophrenia and Schizoaffective Disorder (According to Psycho-pharmacology and Psychopathology)

We have already seen some differences between schizophrenia and schizoaffective disorder in the descriptions of Olanzapine. Here, I will discuss the existence of schizophrenia, and the psycho-pharmacological and psychopathological phenomena.

At first glance, the differences between schizophrenic disorder and schizoaffective disorder, including atypical psychoses, should be clear by virtue of the effects of Olanzapine. In these investigations, it could be clarified whether Olanzapine is effective for schizophrenic disorder or atypical psychoses.

And, at last, indications and actual effects of Olanzapine can be clarified by making a comparative study of clinical pathogenetic states of schizophrenia and schizoaffective disorder including atypical psychoses.

Schizophrenia

Symptoms: Onset is commonly chronic or sub chronic. The fundamental disturbance is an indistinct boundary between self and others. If not treated in the early stages, the prognosis will not always be good. If the disorder is left unattended, pathological experiences develop and become worse and worse. Disturbance of consciousness is rare. Emotional and psychomotor disturbances are found as peripheral symptoms.

Schizoaffective Disorder

Symptoms: Onset is commonly acute and prognosis is good for each occurrence, but the symptoms repeatedly recur. The main symptoms are emotional, consciousness and psychomotor disturbances. Usually, the disorder shows bipolarity, such as manic-depressive disorder, anxiety-ecstasy disorder, and excitement-bewilderment.

Both disorders can be fundamentally defined as integrative disorders in brain, as if these two disorders seem to be undoubtedly different.

On the one hand, it could be said that, with schizoaffective disorders including atypical psychoses, it is as if a lot of dopamine as a neurotransmitter were suddenly injected into A10 nervous nucleus. On the other hand, in schizophrenic disorders, it is as if dopamine were slowly and gradually injected into A10 nucleus over a period of several months.(44)

The former gives rise to sudden destruction of the route from midbrain to amygdaloidal nucleus, hippocampus, basal ganglia, nucleus accumbens and frontal association area, and the A10 nerves, which cause a human being to have a feeling of well being by secretion of dopamine. These phenomena invite self-destruction, which might be experienced as 'world destruction phantasm,' since it is impossible to experience the awareness of self destruction. Instead, these patients experience a peripheral world destruction phantasm, as a projected shadow between self and others.

Concerning these phenomena in the former, we can speculate that the destruction of connective routes to the A10 nerves began at birth, and was complete by adolescence. It has been shown that, in such cases, the first period of rebellion already lacked the stage of individualization, which usually happens at around at age three. As a result, when this child arrives to adolescence, each area of the brain (from midbrain to amygdaloidal nucleus, hippocampus, basal ganglia, nucleus accumbens and frontal association area) has begun to work individually, and were fixed to each other, instead of connecting to A10 nerves.

These phenomena have had an effect on the decision-making of doctors when prescribing medicines. In fact, it will take several months to see the results of medications in schizophrenias, while with schizoaffective disorders, only a few days are required.

From these phenomena, the exact differences between the two disorders have been clarified. Additionally, when symtomatic cross studies were performed, results showed that the two disorders continue to share symptoms. But schizophrenic patients respond to medication very slowly, while those suffering from schizoaffective disorders respond quickly. And while it is supposed that disturbed areas might be similar or the same in both disorders, the former could be irreversible and the latter reversible. In fact, hallucinations and delusions continue for longer and longer periods with schizophrenia, compared with a short recovery time with schizoaffective disorders.

When a pathological experience, such as a hallucination or delusion, was established as a route of 'actual past experiences' in the memory circuit to A10 nerves through Dopamine, it could be too difficult to change memories of these experiences to unrealistic past experiences defined as good feelings, even if Olanzapine makes the effect to A10 through Dopamine. Of course, it is possible that the amount of time that has passed does not affect whether these phenomena are reversible or irreversible. While the midbrain connects to the cerebral limbic lines, which work on emotional responses, it is thought that the functioning of the nervous line is related to hallucination and delusion.

It has been speculated that pathological impulses can be sent via nerves to the limbic line for even a short time (as little as a moment up to several years). This idea was brought to light by the immediate effects of metha-anphetamine on hallucination and delusion. It was further speculated that although hallucination and delusion due to hyperactivity of Dopamine in the midbrain-limbic route produce a pathogenetic state at first, over time, these situation comes to rest as an individual's natural physiological state. These phenomena could be the pathogenetic situations of schizophrenia.

Furthermore, the pathological route of the phenomena spread until the amygdaloidal nucleus, hippocampus, basal ganglia, nucleus accumbens and frontal association areas, and these pathogenetic phenomena were changed to the defense responses, and as a result, each area came to work as an individual self defense response in each area. In a normal human being, the impulse route is originally established by connection of amygdaloidal nucleus, hippocampus, basal ganglia, nucleus accumbens and frontal association area to A10 nerve. But, when—as with the pathologies under discussion—each area begins to work individually, the A10 nerves lose their role of conductor in the brain.

If these pathological conditions become established, the role of the brain would be completely different. Furthermore, as we have seen, when these situations are prolonged, they will cease to be pathological and become, instead, the normal physiology of the individual.

At the beginning of onset, sleep disturbance often occurs, which is probably due to a disturbance of the nucleus accumbens. It is thought that when some disturbance or abnormality occurs in the relationship between A10 nerves and other areas, schizophrenia began to appear. The first sign will be confusion between a state of awakeness and a state of sleep. Along with these phenomena, anger by over secretion of Noradrenalin due to secretive disturbance of catecholamine and fear experiences by over secretion of Adrenalin are transmitted to the cerebral limbic system. As a result, the over-secreted TRH works on the ability to reason, so that an individual can lapse into emotional excitement. Furthermore, pathological nervous roots connect to the hippocampus as a memory circuit, and pathological experiences remain in the memory as the actual experience in spatio-temporal confusion.

It might be defined as schizophrenia that the whole phenomenon has gradually appeared and developed over time, so that neither psychotherapies nor medications are so effective anymore.

In the development of these phenomena, only the A10 nerves are affected by medicine and can therefore improve or pause. Until today, it is speculated that only Olanzapine will work A10 selectively, or only Olanzapine will be effective for schizophrenia.

Schizoaffective disorders appear suddenly, causing acute changes in human brain functioning. Any clinician commonly hears from patients, "I became suddenly confused one day, and from then on, I never am not able to remember on afterward." The complaint showed his onset to be sudden.

But, when a patient complains, "I have been hearing strange voices since last spring or at the beginning of autumn," he will definitely be diagnosed as schizophrenic. Thus, spatiotemporal situations of onset are significantly different between schizophrenia and schizoaffective disorders.

Schizoaffective disorder shows a special feature called "attack" by Kimura, B(45). In the existential structure of epilepsy, he clarified the derivation of the word "epilepsy" to mean a "sudden attack, being caught, and being suppressed." Accompanied with this, Plugge, H., physician, defined the crisis in Attack and Crisis, as a severe and sudden attack accompanied with fear of death and sensation of falling in darkness. Furthermore, since all experience of time is suspended, it is difficult for the patient to explain the exact time of an attack, and sometimes memories disappear. Attack has special properties, too, such as the course of recovery, quitting and improvement or sudden death. Additionally, Attack as crisis shows the interruption of one continuous phenomenon.

Furthermore, von Weiztsaecker, V. asserted that we must stop identifying mental with subjective. An organism without consciousness and an organism without experiencing the special contents are similarly related to the outside world(45) Similarly, Kimura brings his own logic is as follows: the most important point of the psychosomatology of a schizoaffective patient, as differientiated from others' psychosomatology might be that the schizoaffective patient never develops a logical argument of the exterior mental operation. In other words, he never invites the easy or common meaning. The epileptic existential pattern, or constructive moment, is already integrated widely into the existential construction of a normal human being. This limited psychopathological area, especially the group called atypical psychoses or periodic psychoses, is included into the same existential construction. The group is clinically characterized as suffering from a weakness of consciousness.

The differentiation of these pathologies is clarified by the definition of diseases of Heidegger, M. He defined the human existential construction as "life order;" and diseases, which threaten the construction, as "life order crisis." And he argued that all life order crisis is defined as spatiotemporal existence(46). From this perspective, we could define schizophrenia as a situation that develops gradually and slowly, and that retains the individual integrity of each are of the brain. And schizoaffective disorder might be defined as a sudden spatiotemporal attack.

It is possible to that both situations respond to Olanzapine. It is effective for the immediate and dramatic symptoms of schizoaffective disorders, and is also easily effective on the slow and gradual development of schizophrenic disorders.

From these discussions, we can surmise that those who argue for a non-organic, symtomatic and statistical diagnose might be the same contingent who define an organic human being as a nonorganic existence and who treat human beings as nonorganic existences. It is logical that any medicine given in the relationship between a nonorganic patient and therapist will show only nonorganic effects. Only in the clinical situation based on the exact anthropological-psychopathology, it is exactly possible that a human being as an organic existence can absorb a nonorganic medicine into his system to operate as an organic agent

Effects of Olanzapine in Manic and Depressive States

I would like to briefly discuss the effective of Olanzapine on depressive and manic states. However I would never discuss any disease as mono-psychosis. I would have to discuss, rather, each psychosis according to its psychopathological and psychopharmacological makeup. In fact, the real atypical psychosis has been discussed in the same terms as schizoaffective disorder for convenience' sake. But the real atypical psychosis will have to be diagnosed without regard to many of the symptoms and situations of schizoaffective disorders. In other words, schizoaffective disorder was defined without regard to most psychogenetic symptoms, so it is common knowledge that the vast differences between atypical psychosis and schizoaffective disorder actually exist.

Acknowledging the actual existence of a clinical, psychopathological situation called atypical psychosis, schizoaffective disorder actually exists in a different dimension, and are therefore defined differently for diagnostic purposes.

Although atypical psychosis has still not been given an exact diagnostic definition, the exact clinical definition has been clarified as follows (as mentioned above)(3): (a)commonly, the onset of the disease is acute and the prognosis is good for individual occurrences, but the disease has a tendency of recur, (b)the condition of the disease is dominated by emotion, consciousness and psychomotor disorder, (c)the bipolarity in symptoms like manic-depressive, anxiety-trance and excitement-confusion are observed in the course of disease.

Although Lithium derivatives, Valvuloic acid, Na and Carbamazepine had been provided for bipolar disorder, especially the manic state, these medicines never showed much effect. Compared with such a psycho-pharmacological state of affairs, psychopathological studies on manic-depressive illness have appeared one after another, even in Japan.

Ohashi M. has already made the interesting observation that Schneider, K. argued that any motivation to regard a manic state as a single syndrome. He defined a manic state as accompanied by symptoms of inner disquieting and anxiety states.(49) Schilder, P., however, argued that a manic state is defined as the defensive power of conquering unpleasurable experiences and changing them into pleasurable experiences, as a water tank functions: the water level goes up and down. When the water increases by biological energy, water flows out and, as a result, a manic state is invited.

Tellenbach speaks of the appearance of the manic state in terms of the personality of the person. For instance, it has been observed that a melancholia-affinitive cycloid personality falls into a manic state in some special situations, instead of the expected depression. However, Freud, S. argued that a manic state is usually observed when a poor person suddenly becomes rich or when a person is freed from a suppressed situation. And Klein, M. argues the existence of the manic stage as a defense. Thus, the relationships between the manic and depressive states are described in psychopathology, as mentioned above.

Additionally, when there is improvement of pain and fear, the manic defense changes and sometimes a wrong circuit is established, which can interfere with future improvement. Hirose, T. spoke about depression in biological studies. He said that depression is defined as a refractory period accompanied with suppression and conservative withdrawal like hibernation, compared with preparation of the fight made against danger, and anxiety is accompanied by excitement of the autonomic nervous system in the manic state.(49) Additionally, Ohashi, M. classified depressions into the simple type (reactive), the responsible type and the discharged type. And Takahashi, R. clarified depression from the perspective of biological psychiatry(48) as follows: Depression will have to be discussed in terms of the traditional idea called "black bile over secretion theory." But the World Health Organization (WHO) had already classified depressions into the morning depressive type (50%) and the afternoon depressive type (12.5%) in 62.5% circadian rhythmic depressions by use of the classification method of Kielholz, P.

From these observations, we can see evidence that depressions could be a biological pathogenetic situation. After Kielholz, studies of of circadian rhythm in depressive states and in manic-depressive illness have been performed by Middelhoff, H.D.(1967), Waldman, H. (1972) and in manic depressive illness by Hertrich, O., Hirasawa (1966), Waldman, H. (1972) and Takahashi (50). These reports show evidence that the circadian rhythm was present in depression and manic-depressive illness, or short term and long term depressive and manic-depressive disorders. Sleep at night improves neurotic-exhaustion, it is expected that morning depressions are fewer than afternoon depressions due to daytime exhaustion.

But, patients of manic depressive illnesses and simple depressions showed exactly opposite results. From these observations and opinions, an existence of biological disturbances might be suspected in manic depressive illness and depression. Thus, since it was thought that the circadian rhythm was made based on monoamine theory, measurement of tyrosine as pre-amino-acid of catecholamine was performed. It was argued that the serum level of tyrosine showed the lowest level at 10am, and when this state improved, tyrosine rhythm returned to a healthy pattern.(51) At any rate, studies after the measurement of catecholamine will never be shown.

The psychopharmacological studies of Olanzapine as MARTA had direct effects on depression. (Recall that a MARTA is a Multiacting Receptor Targeted Antipsychotic.) It was already described that MARTA, by cutting off the connection between D_2 receptors and 5-HT_2 receptors, improved both positive and negative symptoms. Furthermore, it was clarified that Olanzapine cut off not only the relationship between D_2 receptors and 5-HT_2 receptors, but also the relationships among much of receptors.

Here, I submit that "previous negative symptoms" might be recognized as a depressive state based on the studies and arguments outlined above. The category "positive symptoms" never exists in psychopathology; it exists only in symtomatic and statistical explanations. When the discussion of negative symptoms was brought to the same table, the expression of negative symptoms might be the main existing form of the core of schizophrenia, and same existing form of a depressive state. The form called positive symptoms should be expressed as peripheral symptoms, as compared with core symptoms.(12)-(20)

From these points of view, Kimura, B. argued that the core of schizophrenia should be defined as its form and features; schizophrenia should never be discussed and treated in terms of a basic disease unit. Schizophrenia as a disease is seen as only peripheral symptoms like hallucination and delusion, which is subject to treatment. Olanzapine, by working on the A10 nerves, affects schizophrenia as a life form and feature. The A10 nerves in the tegmentum of the midbrain are connected with midbrain, amygdaloidal nucleus (related to emotion, fear, adaptability), hippocampus, basal ganglia (related to somatic motor), nucleus accumbens (related to limbic system, known as emotional and visceral brain) and frontal association area (related to personality, movement motivation and plan) make human beings aware of pleasure by the secretion of Dopamine. In other word, A10 nerves act in the role of conductor in brain.(29)-(32)

It may therefore be speculated that indications of Olanzapine as MARTA would be included in depressive states. This phenomenon was shown by clinical cases, comparing situations in which Olanzapine was switched to Aripirazol, and the opposite response was elicited. As a result, it was clarified that taking both Olanzapine and Aripirazol was the most effective method.

Furthermore, there are increasing reports that Olanzapine showed significant effectiveness against nausea and vomiting due to anticancer agents(52).

In light of the above, I am hopeful for the expansion of indications in Olanzapine, and I emphatically encourage continued studies of Olanzapine in relation to selective works of the A10 nerves.

Immunological Properties of Olanzapine

Immunologically, Olanzapine has been shown effective both in the elevation of T cell lines and in natural killer-cell activity, in contrast to the seesaw phenomenon in other medicines. Such effectiveness has not been seen in immunological medications previously.

There are many studies available that show antipsychotics and antidepressants like SSRIs cause an elevation of natural killer activity, instead of the reduction of activities of the T-cell line.(53)(54) Thus, in mental disorders, mortality due to viral diseases and cancers have been continuously at the lowest levels, compared with the highest levels of bacterial infections.(53)

It had been well known that the T-cell line performs killer-cell action only against encountered enemies like bacteria that have been met previously and disturb a host. But natural killer cells kill and destroy whole non-self species, unrelated to the previous or the first encounters.

Until now, it has been thought that immune abilities with both characteristics were not possible. But, it is now speculated that Olanzapine could have both immune abilities since Olanzapine has showed the activation of both T-cell line and natural killer cells. From these results, it looks hopeful that Olanzapine could elicit an immune response in the host against not only invaders but also inner enemies.

VI. Conclusion

Retrospective studies were conducted on 453 cases who were prescribed Olanzapine in the author's clinic. The following phenomena were indicated:

1. Possibilities of expansion of indications as MARTA.
2. Necessity of psychopathological studies based on A10 nerve works.
3. Evaluation of takin g both Olanzapine and Aripirazol, instead of switching effects.
4. Unusual and special immune responses against both virus and bacteria, and cancer.
5. Significant elevation of quality-of-life due to the reduction of side effects of anti-cancer agents.

It was shown that Olanzapine was effective for not only schizophrenia and its peripheral disorders based on the symptomatolocial diagnostic manuals, but also had much potential for other disorders. And regarding the A10 nerve function, it was shown that Olanzapine significantly improved numerous cases of integration disturbances in the brain.

When Olanzapine was first clinically prescribed, it was necessary to test and study psychopathological results before treating Olanzapine as an organic medicine. Otherwise, symtomatic and statistical diagnostic practices would be denied.

Of course, it would be inevitable that Olanzapine has side effects, since it is man made, but it was shown that some of the side effects of Olanzapine were precisely the intended effects of some other medications, for example, antiviral and anticancer effects in SSRIs and SNRIs.

Olanzapine seemed to be among the strongest medicines for human beings, but showed gentle effects in both low and high dosages in the context of psychotherapy.(55)(56)

I am skeptical about the validity of the results of testing antipsychotic medicines on animals, since there is a vast difference between the workings of the brains of animals and humans beings.(And, in my opinion, the human being is not necessarily the highest of the organisms.) In some such studies, Olanzapine was added Fluoxetine, but it is difficult to understand to what purpose.(57)

I am emphatically in favor of deep and thorough testing of new medicines before introducing the medication at large. I am not a proponent of mono-medicine prescriptions as a general rule, but it was important to learn the potential of Olanzapine, a drug that showed much promise. I, therefore, introduced the retrospective studies on Olanzapine to know the details of its effects, both alone and in switching and in combination with other medications, and because I have profound doubts about the accuracy of symtomatic and statistical clinical diagnostic and prescriptive style.

Furthermore, no psychopathological research has been available in contemporary clinical studies, although organic human beings have treated organic patients by use of organic psychotherapies. I recognize that organic treatments have gone out of favor by decree of symtomatic and statistical diagnostic manuals. In this diagnostic and treatment atmosphere, although organic therapists should treat patients as organic entities by use of organic medicines, all clinicians have had to forget about such a style.

Thus, when I investigated the detailed effects of Olanzapine, I discovered how to treat the medicine as organic substance, because Olanzapine showed a number of organic effects, even on young children.

And, finally, I believe that the practice of psychiatry has been virtually destroyed by the introduction of the symtomatic and statistical fundamental philosophy.

As clinicians, we must continue to treat our patients as living human beings.

Acknowledgements

First, I must describe this book is the psychiatric history of clients, who willingly participated in the project. I would like to express my appreciation to these clients with a full heart and a promise to never forget their kind cooperation.

Further, I wish to acknowledge the work of a number of psychiatrists who taught psychopathology and psychopharmacology kindly and gently from 1973, with hope for their eternal health. I will never forget their strong guidance and deep philosophy.

In particular, I wish to thank Mr. Hiroki Mizutani, who tirelessly analyzed much of the data in the studies described in this book.

And, finally, I would like to express appreciation to the medical employees who promote organic and living medicines.

Hajime Jozuka, M.D.,
Jozuka Mental Clinic
April, 2010.

References

(1) American Psychiatric Association: DSM-III. Diagnostic and Statistical Manual of Mental Disorders. 3rd. Ed.The Association, Washinton,D.C. 1980.
(2) Pauleikhoff, B: Atypische Psychosen. S.Karger, Basel, 1957.
(3) Hatotani, T. (author and editor). *Internal Secretion Psychiatry*, Igaku-shoin, P.218, 1978.
(4) Kimura, B., *Self, Distance and Time* (Phenomenological Psychopathology) Kobundo, Tokyo, Japan, 1981.
(5) Fink, JS, Smith, GP, "Mesolimbicocortical dopamine terminal fields are necessary for normal locomotor and investigatory exploration in rats", Brain Res. 1980 Oct. 20;199(2):359-84.
(6) Lembreghts, M, Ansseau, M:, "Biological markers in schizophrenia", Enchephale, 1993 Sep-Oct;19(5):501-23.
(7) Crescimanno G, Sorbera F, Emmi A, Amato G.,"Inhibitory effect of A10 dopaminergic neurons of the ventral tegmental area on the orienting response evoked by acoustic stimulation in the cat". Brain Res. Bull. 1998;45(1)61-5.
(8) S Miyamoto, GE Duncan, CE Marx, JA Lieberman, "Treatments for schizophrenia: a critical review of pharmacology and mechanisms of action of antipsychotic drugs", Molecular Psychiatry, 10, 79–104. 2005,
(9) Harada, K. (Ed.), *Symptomatic Psychoses*. Kokusai Pub. 1978.
(10) Selye, H., *Stress*. Acta. Montoreal, 1950.
(11) Tellenbach, H., *Melancholie*, Springer-Verlag Berlin/Heidelberg 1961, 1974 und 1976.
(12) Doi, T. (Ed.): Psychopathology on Schizophrenia 1. Tokyo Univ. Pub. 1972.
(13) Miyaoto, T.(Ed.), "Psychopathology on Schizophrenia 2", Tokyo Univ. Pub. 1974.
(14) Kimura, B.(Ed.), "Psychopathology on Schizophrenia 3", Tokyo Univ. Pub. 1974.
(15) Ogino, K. (Ed.), "Psychopathology on Schizophrenia 4", Tokyo Univ. Pub. 1976.
(16) Kasahara, Y. (Ed.), "Psychopathology on Schizophrenia 5", Tokyo Univ. Pub.1977.
(17) Yasunaga, H. (Ed.), "Psychopathology on Schizophrenia 6", Tokyo Univ. Pub. 1978.
(18) Yuasa, S. (Ed.), "Psychopathology on Schizophrenia 7", Tokyo Univ. Pub. 1979.

(19) Nakai, H. (Ed.), "Psychopathology on Schizophrenia 8", Tokyo Univ. Pub. 1979.
(20) Kawakubo, Y. (Ed.), "Psychopathology on Schizophrenia 9", Tokyo Univ. Pub. 1980
(21) Heidegger, M.: *Being and Time* (translated from Sein und Zeit). State University of New York Pr.1996.
(22) Heidegger, M., Boss, M. et al.: Zollikon Seminars, Protocols, Conversations, Letters, Northwestern University Press. US. 2000.
(23) Heidegger, M., *Existential Foundation of Medicine and Psychology*. Jason Aronson; New Edition, 1995.
(24) von Weizsaecker, V. *Studien zur Pathogenese*, Thieme, Wiesbaden, 1946.
(25) Boss, M.: Psychoanalysis and Daseinsanalysis. Basic Books, 1963.
(26) Kimura, B.: Zuwischen Mensch und Mensch. Wissenschaftlische Buchengesellschaft.
(27) Zutt,J und C. Kulenkampff: "Die paranoide Syndrom in anthropologischer Sicht." Berlin Goettingen-Heiderberg, 1959.
(28) Penfield, W. : *The Mystery of The Mind*. Princeton University Press New York, 1975.
(29) Matsushima, Y., Matsuda, T., Narita, M. et al., "The Study of Drug Dependence" (No.432): Ventral Tegmentum—Activity of Dopamine Nerve by Opioid. J. Japan Pharmacology Assoc. vol. 128, page13 − 13: 2008.
(30) Saeki, Y., Aiyama, K.: "Antipsychotics in Newage—variation and pharmacological effects". Daily Life, page16 − 20 : 2001。
(31) Bymaster, F.P. 、Nakazawa, T.: Pharmacological Fundation of Olanzapine in MARTA line antipsychotics. Clin. Pharm. Vol.2,-8, 885 − 911, 1999.
(32) Marsh, E. Stockton, B.S. and Kurt Rasmussen: "Electrophysiological Effect of Olanzapine, a Novel Atypical Antipsychotic, on A9 and A10 Dopamine Neurons". Neuropsychopharmacology 14-2, 97-104: 1996.
(33) Nozawa, K., Sekine, A., Hozumi, T. Shimizu, T.m "Effect of Olanzapine for Residual Symptoms of Melancholia Affinitive Major Depression". Psychiat. Therapeutics 24(7): 859-866、2009.
(34) Blenner, C., *An Elementary Treatment of Psychoanalysis*, 1955.
(35) Stahl, S.M.: Essential Psychopharmacology; The Prescriber's Guide. New York. NY: Cambridge UP: 2004.
(36) Zanarini MC, Frankenburg FR: Olanzapine treatment of female borderline personality disorder patients: a double-blind, placebo-controlled pilot study. J Clin Psychiatry 62(11):849-54. (2001)
(37) Zanarini MC, Frankenburg FR, Parachini EA: A preliminary, randomized trial of fluoxetine, olanzapine, and the olanzapine-fluoxetine combination in women with borderline personality disorder. J Clin Psychiatry 65(7):903-7. (2004), Kato, M., Hozaki, H. (ed.), *Psychiatric Dictionary*, Kobundo,1993.

(38) Pierre V. T., Frank, P. Bymaster, Nick, Tye: Olanzapine: A Novel Antipsychotic. M17; Seiichi Matsumoto(ed.): Sexuality and Human Bonding. Exerpta Medica. Elsevier, 1996.(12th World Congress of Sexology, Tokyo, Japan).
(39) American Psychiatric Association: *Diagnostic and Statistical Manual of Medical Disorder IV*:1994.
(40) Jozuka, H.: *From Conception to Adolescence*, Bibliobooks, Israel, 2006.
(41) Boss、M., *Psychoanalysis and Daseinsanalysis*. Basic Books, 1963.
(42) Heidegger, M., Boss, M. et al., :Zollikon Seminars Protocols- conversations-letters. Northwestern University Press, U.S. 2000.
(43) Jozuka, H., "Clinical Indication of Sulpiride: Psychopathological discussion of depressions", Consultation and New Medicines. Vol.18(10)、139-146 : 1981
(44) Ganong, W.F., *Medical Physiology*. Maruzen.1988
(45) Kimura, B. (ed.), *Antholopology of Epilepsy—Existential Construction*.Tokyo Univ. Press. 1980
(45) Weizsaecker, V. von: Der Gestaltkreis. Theorie der Einheit von Wahrnehmen und Bewegen. Thieme, Stuttgart 1940.
(46) Heidegger, M., Sein und Zeit. Sevensedition, Neomarius Verlag, Tubingen, 1962. (Translated by John Macquarrie and Edward Robinson: Being and Time. Harper Collins Publishers, 10 East St., NY:10022: 1962.
(47) Kasahara, Y.(ed.), Psychopathology of manic depressive illness 1. Kobundo, Tokyo,1976
(48) Miyamoto, T. (ed.), Psychopathology of manic depressive illness 2. Kobundo, Tokyo,1977.
(49) Iida, S. (ed.), Psychopathology of manic depressive illness 3. Kobundo, Tokyo,1979
(50) Waldman, H., Die Tagesschwankung in der Depression als thythmisches Phaenomen. Fortschr. Neurol. Psychiat. 40: 83, 1972.
(51) Klempel, K.: Orientierende Untersuchung des zirkabidianen Plasma-Tyrosin-Rhythmus depressiver Syndrom, Unterschiedliche Atiologie, Arch, Psychiat. Mervankr. 216:131, 1972.
(52) Tan L, Liu J, Liu X, Chen J, Yan Z, Yang H, Zhang D, Clinical research of Olanzapine for prevention of chemotherapy-induced nausea and vomiting, J Exp Clin Cancer Res. 2009 Sep 23;28:131.
(53) Jozuka, H., *Introduction to Psychoneuroimmunopathology and Clinical Practice*. Bibliobooks, Israel:2004.
(54) Jozuka, H., Psychoneuroimmunopathology & Daseinsanalysis, Bibliobooks, Israel, 2008.
(55) Nakai, H., *The Last Lecture ̄Schizophrenia*, Misuzu, Tokyo, 1998.
(56) Shirakawa, O., "Treatment of Bipolar disorder by atypical antipsychotics", Psychotherapeutics, vol. 20：1239–1246：2005

(57) Zhang, W. et al.: Synergistic Effects of Olanzapine and other antipsychotic agents in combination with Fluoxetine on Norepinephrine and Dopamine Release in Rat Prefrontal Cortex. Neuropsychopharmacology, 23, (3): 2000.
(58) Lieb K, Völlm B, Rücker G, Timmer A, Stoffers JM.:Pharmacotherapy for borderline personality disorder: Cochrane systematic review of randomised trials. Br J Psychiatry. Jan;196(1):4-12.2010.
(59) Bellino S, Paradiso E, Bogetto F.:Efficacy and tolerability of pharmacotherapies for borderline personality disorder.CNS Drugs. 22(8):671-92. Review.2008.
(60) Linehan MM, McDavid JD, Brown MZ, Sayrs JH, Gallop RJ.: Olanzapine plus dialectical behavior therapy for women with high irritability who meet criteria for borderline personality disorder: a double-blind, placebo-controlled pilot study. J Clin. Psychiatry. 69(6):999-1005, 2008.
(61) Abraham PF, Calabrese JR.:Evidenced-based pharmacologic treatment of borderline personality disorder: a shift from SSRIs to anticonvulsants and atypical antipsychotics. J Affect Disord. 111(1):21-30. Epub 2008 Mar 4. Review, 2008.
(62) Damsa C, Adam E, De Gregorio F, Cailhol L, Lejeune J, Lazignac C, Allen MH. :Intramuscular olanzapine in patients with borderline personality disorder: an observational study in an emergency room. Gen Hosp Psychiatry. 29(1):51-3, 2007.
(63) Shoja-Shafti S. :Treatment of borderline personality disorder with olanzapine. Arch Iran Med. 9(4):403-5, 2006.
(64) Pascual JC, Madre M, Soler J, Barrachina J, Campins MJ, Alvarez E, Pérez V. :Injectable atypical antipsychotics for agitation in borderline personality disorder. Pharmacopsychiatry. 39(3):117-8, 2006.
(65) Galinowski A.:[Borderline personality disorder] Encephale. 31 Pt 2:S73-5. French. No abstract available, 2005.
(66) Soler J, Pascual JC, Campins J, Barrachina J, Puigdemont D, Alvarez E, Pérez V. :Double-blind, placebo-controlled study of dialectical behavior therapy plus olanzapine for borderline personality disorder. Am J Psychiatry. 2005 Jun;162(6):1221-4. Erratum in: Am J Psychiatry. 2008 Jun;165(6):777.
(67) Bogenschutz MP, George Nurnberg H.: Olanzapine versus placebo in the treatment of borderline personality disorder. J Clin Psychiatry. 65(1):104-9,2004.

Epilogue

When I observe our society, I see a sudden rise of borderline personality disorders and many miserable problems for many people as a result.

And when I look around, I also see rapid growth of economy one minute, and an economic slump the next minute, all because of the variations of the markets in the big countries; I see big companies claim to be in economic crises in order to get into step with ally countries (even though they are actually operating in surplus); I see increased layoffs. And I see companies attaching great importance to production, but forgetting about the basic human needs of their employees, and executives.

Made in the USA
Monee, IL
04 November 2026

67377477R10059